Essential Oils for Dogs:

The Complete Guide to Safe and Simple Ways to Use Essential Oils for a Happier, Relaxed and Healthier Dog

(Includes Essential Oil Recipes)

BY: Julie Summers

Copyright © 2016 Julie Summers

All rights reserved.

This book is or any part of it may not be reproduced in any written, electronic, recording, or photocopying without written permission of the publisher or author having intellectual rights over the content of the book. The exception would be in the case of brief quotations embodied in the critical articles or reviews and pages where permission is specifically granted by the publisher or author.

Although every precaution has been taken to verify the accuracy of the information contained herein, the author and publisher assume no responsibility for any errors or omissions. No liability is assumed for any damage or damages that may result from the use of information contained herein.

Information contains in this book in solely for information purposes and does not intend in any way to replace professional medical and health advices rendered by practitioners in the field of veterinary medicine and you are further recommended to seek professional advice before using this material.

ISBN-10: 197616401X
ISBN-13: 978-1976164019

CONTENTS

	Introduction	i
1	What are Essential Oils?	1
2	Do Essential Oils Work for Dogs?	13
3	The Basics of Essential Oils for Dogs	32
4	How to Safely use Essential Oils for you Dog	45
5	Precautions and Safety in Using Essential Oils	55
6	Essential Oil Recipes	65
7	Conclusion	97

INTRODUCTION

Essential oils have previously been used for enhancement of well-being in humans but, are they safe to use on animals and pets, particularly on dogs that have been proven to be loyal companions of people?

The holistic approach to the use of essential oils for dogs is now gaining popularity among pet and dog lovers but misinformation has also taken its toll on some who were misguided in the proper ways of using essential oils on dogs. Through this eBook, we aim to correct this misinformation and provide you with a safe and easy to follow guide you can use while applying essential oils to your dog.

In this eBook, "Essential Oils for Dogs: The Complete Guide to Safe and Simple Ways to Use Essential Oils for a Happier, Relaxed and Healthier Dog complete with Essential Oil Recipes for Aromatherapy Natural Dog Care Remedies", you can expect a thorough understanding of essential oils on dogs including its various applications, benefits, safety precautions and uses plus, added homemade recipes which are sure to help you minimize your budget while maintaining your dog's health and well-being.

Through this guide, you can provide your pet the essential care he needs to improve his health condition, stabilize his mental and emotional state and improve his behavior.

This holistic approach to aromatherapy is geared towards enhancing the total well-being of your dog and likewise, developing a stronger bond between the two of you.

WHAT ARE ESSENTIAL OILS

An essential oil is an organic compound substance taken from the sac, glandular hair and in any other parts of the plants including leaves, roots, seeds, fruit or flowers. They are the essence of that particular plant and are responsible for the unique scent of that specific plant. An essential oil is volatile and therefore evaporates easily in addition to being diffusible.

Essential oils need to be diluted before each use as they are highly concentrated. Each essential oil carries individual properties like color, scent, healing effects and other chemical properties.

Many of these essential oils are

antibacterial, antifungal, antiviral, antioxidant and anti-inflammatory. They also affect the emotional function of the body by stimulating particular areas of the brain and can even be a sedative.

When you extract essential oils from plants through steam distillation, you can produce hydrosol, a water-based substance, which is a by-product obtained from the initial process. Hydrosol contains only a little part of the essential oil and a large part of the water-soluble parts of the plants. Unlike essential oils which are highly concentrated, hydrosol is not concentrated and can be used undiluted. You can also add essential oils for a combined effect.

For a highly sensitive dog, you can have hydrosol as an alternative option from using essential oils.

How are Essential Oil Made?

To extract a plant's essential oil, you may use the following methods:

- Steam Distillation
- Solvent Extraction

- Carbon Dioxide Extraction
- Manual Extraction

Distillation

The majority of essential oils are produced by the process of distillation. In distillation, water is heated to produce steam, which carries the most volatile substance of the scent. Then the steam is chilled in a condenser and the distilled result is collected. Normally, the essential oil is lighter and so it floats on top of the hydrosol, which is the distilled water component. Later, you will be working on separating the two compound elements.

Steam Distillation
Steam distillation uses an external source of steam, which carries the steam through the pipes into the distillation unit, sometimes at high pressure. Then the steam will pass through the aromatic material and exit into the condenser.

Hydrodistillation
The part of the plant which is used for oil extraction is fully submerged in water, producing the "soup". When steamed, it

contains the essential oil or essence. This process is the oldest method and yet the most versatile and is used in primitive countries. However, there is a risk in this method as the distiller can dry up or overheat giving the essence a burnt smell.

Hydrodistillation works best with powders like spice powders, ground wood and many other tough parts of the plants like the roots as well as other hard materials such as nuts.

Water and Steam Distillation
This method is best for distilling leafy materials but is not applicable for seeds, wood, or roots.

In this method, the leaves are placed in a steamer basket over boiling water, exposing it to the rising steam vapors.

Solvent Extraction

Some flowers used for essential oils like Jasmine and Linden blossom are too delicate to survive the process of distillation. To be able to capture their essence, the process of solvent extraction is used. The blossoms are placed in perforated trays and loaded into an extracting unit. The blossoms are then washed repeatedly using a solvent, usually hexane.

The solution dissolves all the extracted materials which include non-essence wax, highly volatile essential oil and pigments. The solution, with all these dissolvable plant materials and the solvent, is then filtered.

The filtration process is done by subjecting the whole solution to low process distillation to recover the solvent for reuse. The remaining materials that are wax-like are called the concrete and contain as much as 55% of the volatile oil.

To dilute the pure essential oils, it is again processed to remove the wax-like material. To separate the wax; it is warmed and mixed with ethanol alcohol. It is during the heating and stirring process that the concrete is broken up into small globules.

Along with the essence, some wax is also dissolved and can only be removed by freezing the solution at a very low temperature or around 30 degrees Fahrenheit. This way, the wax is separated. As a final precaution, the pure essence is now filtered and declared absolute. This extraction process actually yields three products that you can use. One is the concrete used for solid perfumes, the pure essential oil and the floral waxes which are used as additives to candles, thickening creams and lotions as an alternative to beeswax.

Carbon Dioxide Extraction

When Carbon Dioxide (CO_2) is exposed to high pressure, it changes into liquid form. Its liquid form can be chemically inactive and safe which can then be used to extract the aromatic molecules in a process akin to how the absolutes are extracted. With this process, there will be no traces of solvent residues because CO_2 is again exposed to normal pressure and temperature. It will only revert to its gaseous form and evaporate.

Cold Pressing

Notice that when you score or zest the skin of an orange, you get to see the spray of its essential oil. In the process of cold pressing, machines are able to do just this way. They can mass-produce citrus oils by doing the same procedure—scoring the rinds and capturing the oil that comes out of them. While citrus oils can also be produced through the steam distillation process, the result seems to be of lower quality compared to the ones produced by cold pressing.

Florasols or Phytonic Process

Florasol or phytol process is the newest method used in extracting essential oils by utilizing non-CFS (non-chlorofluorocarbons) as solvents. The oils are called phytols, hence the name of the method it stands for. The unique properties of these solvents were recognized for use in food, aromatherapy, perfume and pharmaceutical industries. Florasol actually comes from the name of the solvent from which it was taken.

Extraction occurs below surrounding temperature level, so there is no occurrence of degradation of the product. The extraction process also uses selective solvents and produces free flowing clear oil, free of waxes.

Brief History of Essential Oils

Essential oils have been around for many centuries and are known to be largely associated with anointing. Throughout history, essential oils were known to be beneficial to health.

Although essential oils have been around for many centuries and their use has been accepted by many around the world, there are still a lot of people who are not aware of their proper use. In fact, many people today, even at this age where everyone has easy and direct access to information, still are misinformed with how to safely use essential oils.

We are also living in an era where maintaining or taking care of our dogs properly has become a luxury only the rich can afford. Our loyal companions are seeing an increasingly long list of health issues due to modern chemicals. As a result of this, veterinary services are getting costly. All these can cause one's budget to soar up.

In an attempt to bring the cost to a level, many resort to using essential oils on dogs. People find them less expensive and better home remedies. The holistic approach of aromatherapy has become popular and more people are gaining interest in its application to animals, particularly dogs.

However, some issues regarding its safety to dogs have arisen as there are cases of negative effects resulting from the use of some essential oils. Before we deal with some of these issues, let's have a brief study on the history of essential oils and how people discovered their uses and integrated them in our health and life!

Ancient Egypt

As early as Ancient Egypt, essential oils were used for cleansing rituals and embalming of their dead as well as mummifying procedures the Egyptians have become famous for doing.

Egyptians were also known for their

knowledge of cosmetology, ointments and aromatic oils. The most famous among their herbal concoctions, "Kyphi" was a mixture of 16 ingredients that were used as incense, medicine or perfume.

At the peak of the Egyptian reign, only their priests were granted access to aromatic oils, being regarded as essential to their union with their gods.

Each deity was dedicated with a specific fragrance and followers would anoint their statues with the essential oils. The pharaoh had his own concoction of specialty blends for meditation, war, love, etc.

Cedar and myrrh were known to be used by Egyptians in their embalming methods and mummification. Traces of these aromatic gums were found in some mummified bodies. Despite the great demand for essential oils, Egyptians never distilled their own and instead preferred to import essential oils.

France

It was in Dordogne region in France where the earliest evidence of human's awareness of the healing properties of plants was found.

In a cave, paintings were drawn in walls which suggested that people were exposed to the use of medicinal herbs as early as 18000 B. C.

China

In China, it was between 2697-2597 B. C. during the reign of Huang Ti, the legendary "Yellow Emperor" was first recorded. The famous book of the emperor, "The Yellow Emperor's book of Internal Medicine" contained the different uses of aromatics which until today are considered useful by practitioners of Eastern Medicine.

India

"Ayur-Veda", the traditional Indian medicine is told to have incorporated essential oils in their healing potions for 3000 years of history. Vedic literature had included more than 700 substances including ginger, cinnamon, sandalwood and myrrh as effective ingredients for healing.

Famous people including Hippocrates, who is known to be the Father of Medicine; Roman emperor, Napoleon Bonaparte; the

Arabian developers of distillations and European crusaders were all linked up to the history of essential oils.

History clearly provided evidence showing that the use of essential oils was more acceptable to people of ancient times and that they were more knowledgeable and exposed to their uses compared to us today.

Historical writings specifically described and illustrated how essential oils, spices, and herbs were used in ancient times. A medical scroll which dated back to 1500 B.C. called "The Ebers Papyrus" was discovered in 1817 and contained over 800 remedies from herbs. To sum it all up, essential oils were used for the following reasons.

- Physical Body Support/Health Improvement and Treatment
- Religious rituals and practices.
- Spiritual Enhancement

It was during the Dark Ages when knowledge and use of essential oils and herbs were curtailed after being associated with practices of witchcraft and sorcery.

The Rediscovery

It was only in the early 20th century when people once again rediscovered essential oils. During the First World War, Dr. Monciere of France used essential oils for the treatment of injured soldiers in the war.

In 1907, Dr. Rene-Maurice Gattefosse, a French chemist, known to many as the Father of Aromatherapy wrote a book entitled "Aromatherapy" which was published in 1937.

Another physician from Paris, Dr. Jean Valnet used essential oils on patients during World War II. Two of Dr. Valnet's students became interested oils and found out about the amazing capabilities of essential oils.

From that time onwards, essential oils were once again accepted and recognized by people in all parts of the world.

DO ESSENTIAL OILS WORK FOR DOGS?

Since essential oils are highly concentrated, they can, therefore, be extremely potent. If you intend to use essential oils on your dogs, be sure to keep them in small dosages and concentration to avoid overdose and negative effects. Always dilute essential oils with carrier oils like olive oil, sweet almond oil, etc. before using any of them on your pet.

With safe essential oils in their diluted form, they are perfectly safe to use on your dogs. They have effective therapeutic value. They can be used as treatments for a great number of ailments ranging from ear and skin infections, allergies, insect bites and rashes to more serious ones like arthritis and even cancer.

Here are some of the benefits that you need to know and which you can use while taking care of your dog. Having the right knowledge and the right application on these essential oils will benefit you as well.

Essential Oils are Convenient to Use

Essential oils can be found anywhere today. Because of this gain in popularity, you can easily buy your desired essential oils in malls, specialty stores and even in convenient stores. They come in different kinds and forms. You can find them abounding on the internet and there are lots of websites that offer a free consultation regarding their proper uses. All you have to do is make a search on the kind of need you have before using essential oils.

Essential oils are quick and easy to use and you can have them during the day. If there is something wrong with your pet and you are knowledgeable in using essential oils, you won't find it hard to have your dog ingest his cure. Like people, dogs hate the taste of drugs, too. Simply diffuse an essential oil in your home and you can easily feel its effect on your dog. Essential oils can be found in the form of sprays, rubs, dips, rinse, etc. So all you have to do is find the right one that suits your dog's needs and you can live conveniently with essential oils being handy in your home.

Essential Oils Supports the Body

Essential oils normally support the body and help your dog to have a healthy and strong immune system. They also work on your pet's digestive system. Peppermint oil is effective in soothing digestion.

Essential oils are found to be homeostatic, meaning; they can help maintain a state of equilibrium within the body due to their complex nature. Every essential oil has multiple components which can also produce multiple effects on your dog. Nonetheless, essential oils do not disturb the natural and normal balance of the body. On the other hand, pharmaceutical drugs are literally designed to disrupt the body's homeostasis because of their natural components which are synthetic chemicals.

Essential Oils Works on your Dog's Emotions

The benefits of essential oils include penetrating the part of the brain which is responsible for emotions, survival instincts and memory. This is the reason why using some essential oils can provide calming effects to your dog and soothe his senses when he is angry, stressed or suffering from anxiety.

Soothes Muscle Discomfort

By using essential oils, you can help your dog get relief from some muscle strain or discomfort. They can be massaged or diffused to give him a soothing effect.

Benefits of Oil Essentials to Body System

Cardiovascular System

Body Parts:

Blood, blood vessels, heart, veins, arteries, and capillaries.

Essential Oils:

Helichrysum, Lavender, Lemon, Orange, Ylang Ylang, Jasmine Absolute, Joy, Peace & Calming, Citrus Fresh, Joy, EndoFlex, Copaiba.

Digestive System

Body Parts:

Mouth, tongue, teeth, intestines, liver, salivary glands, pharynx, gallbladder, pancreas, stomach, appendix, esophagus, anal canal, rectum.

Essential Oils:

Lemon, Orange, Ylang Ylang, Peppermint,

Thieves, EndoFlex, Purification, AromaEase, Frankincense, Blue Cypress, Tangerine, DiGize, Spearmint, Ginger, TummyGize.

Endocrine System

Body Parts:

The pituitary gland, pineal gland, adrenals, testes, thyroid gland, ovaries, parathyroids, pancreas, thymus and hypothalamus.

Essential Oils:

Helichrysum, Spearmint, Frankincense, Myrrh, Jasmine Absolute, Lavender, Clary Sage, EndoFlex, En-R-Gee, Thieves, Valor.

Immune System

Body Parts:

Portions of many different systems that fight diseases via the anatomic, inflammatory and immune responses.

Essential Oils:

Eucalyptus Blue, En-R-Gee, Helichrysum,

Citrus Fresh, Tangerine, Thieves, ComforTone, Abundance, Lemon, Lemongrass, Hinoki, Frankincense, Cumin, Orange, Myrrh, Lavender, Breathe Again, EndoFlex, Lime, Ravintsara, Stress Away.

Integumentary System

Body **Parts**:

Nails, skin, hair, sense receptors, oil glands, and sweat glands.

Essential Oils:

Lavender, Frankincense, Geranium, Peppermint, Lemon, Thieves, Citrus Fresh, Copaiba, Purification, Orange, Jasmine Absolute, Manuka, Clary Sage, Ylang Ylang, Gentle Baby, Melissa, Melrose, Myrrh, Patchouli, Rose, Helichrysum, Sandalwood, Valor.

Limbic System

Body Parts:

Memories, Basic emotions, basic drives,

hippocampus, hypothalamus, and amygdala.

Essential Oils:

Lemon, Copaiba, Lavender, Frankincense, Purification, Peppermint.

Lymphatic System

Body Parts:

Lymph, Lymph nodes, lymphatic vessels, spleen, tonsils, and thymus.

Essential Oils:

Frankincense, Lavender, Lemon, R.C., Thieves, Citrus Fresh, Lemongrass, Orange.

Muscular System

Body Parts:

Skeletal muscles, smooth muscles, cardiac muscles.

Essential Oils:

Frankincense, Idaho Balsam Fir, Orange, Lavender, Myrrh, PanAway, Peace & Calming,

Helichrysum, Deep Relief, Peppermint, Copaiba, Lemongrass, and Spearmint.

Nervous System

Body Parts:

Brain, spinal cord, nerves, brainstem, sensory organs.

Essential Oils:

Lavender, Frankincense, Helichrysum, Myrrh, Peppermint, Valor, Peace & Calming, Copaiba, PanAway.

Reproductive System

Body Parts:

Testes, penis, vas deferens, prostate, urethra, scrotum for the male and for the female, uterus, ovaries, vagina, uterine tubes, mammary glands, and vulva.

Essential Oils:

Ylang Ylang, Frankincense, Lavender, Myrrh,

Orange, Lemon, Jasmine Absolute, Clary Sage, Thieves, EndoFlex.

Respiratory System

Body Parts:

Nose, pharynx, larynx, trachea, bronchi, lungs.

Essential Oils:

Lavender, Idaho Balsam Fir, Helichrysum, Spearmint, Thieves, Purification, Breathe Again, Peppermint, Copaiba, Lemon, R.C., Idaho Blue Spruce, Frankincense, Cedarwood, Eucalyptus, Aroma Siez.

Skeletal System

Body Parts:

Bones, marrow, cartilage, joints.

Essential Oils:

Helichrysum, Peppermint, Idaho Balsam Fir, Clove, Peace & Calming, PanAway, Copaiba, Lemongrass, Deep Relief, Progessence,

Sandalwood.

Urinary System

Body Parts:

Kidneys, ureters, bladder, urethra.

Essential Oils:

Myrrh, Tangerine, Helichrysum, Clove, Lemon, Idaho Balsam Fir, EndoFlex, Purification, Thieves.

Essential Oils that are Safe to Use

Lavender:

- You can use this universal or "must have" oil in its pure state or diluted form.
- Aside from being gentle and soothing, this essential oil is antibacterial, anti-itch, and nerve-calming.
- It is helpful in conditioning your dog to a safe space.
  It can also help to relieve him from skin irritations, allergies, burns, ulcers, car sickness or anxiety and insomnia.

Fennel:

- Use to assist the adrenal cortex and helps release toxins and fluids in tissues.
- It is also helpful in balancing pituitary, pineal, and thyroid glands.

Frankincense:

- Boosts your pet's immune system and has helped in some cases of cancer in humans.
- It can help reduced tumors and external ulcers as well as increase blood supply to the brain.
  Nonetheless, it can also worsen hypertension, so use this with extra caution.

Cardamom:

- Use to normalize appetite, colic, nausea, coughs, and heartburns.
- It is also antibacterial and a diuretic.

Helichrysum:

- This is antibacterial and helps reduce bleeding in injury. It also helps repair nerves, regenerate skin and also useful in cardiovascular diseases.
- Excellent for skin irritations like eczema and effective for healing scars and bruises.

- Anti-inflammatory, analgesic, regenerative and extremely therapeutic.

Spearmint:

- If you need to reduce your dog's weight, this is helpful and it is good for colic, diarrhea, nausea.
- It also helps balance metabolism and stimulates gallbladder.

Bergamot:

- Treatment of ear infection caused by yeast or bacterial overgrowth. Antifungal and soothing.
- Caution: Avoid the sun after use. It can cause photosensitization.

Carrot Seed:

- Perfect for dry, flaky, and sensitive skin prone to infection.
- It is anti-inflammatory, tonic, with moderate antibacterial effects.

- It can also rejuvenate tissue and stimulate regeneration.
- Effective for scar healing.

Cedarwood:

- Good for skin and coat conditioning.
- Treat dermatitis of all types, and flea repellant.
- Antiseptic, circulation-stimulating, and toning.

German Chamomile:

- Good for skin irritations, allergic reactions, burns.

Roman Chamomile:

- Good for soothing the central nervous system.
- Effective for relief of muscle pain.
- Antispasmodic, analgesic, and nerve-calming.

Clary Sage:

- Nerve-calming and gentle when used in small dosage and properly.

Eucalyptus Radiata:

- Good for the relief of chest congestion and effective flea repellant.
- Anti-inflammatory, antiviral, and works as an expectorant.

Geranium:

- Good for skin irritations and fungal ear irritations
- Effective in repelling ticks.
- Gentle and safe antifungal.

Ginger:

- Best for motion sickness and aids in digestion.
- Effective for pain relief caused by arthritis, dysplasia, strains and sprains.

Non-toxic, non-irritating and safe for use is small dosage when properly diluted.

Sweet Marjoram:

- Good for skin infections, wound care and insect repellant.
- Strong antibacterial, with calming effect and muscle relaxant.

Niaouli:

- Good for an ear infection and skin allergies.
- With powerful bacterial properties, Antihistaminic, and less likely to cause irritation than tea tree.

Peppermint:

- Good for arthritis, dysplasia, sprains, and strains.
- Antispasmodic, insect-repellant, and stimulates blood circulation.

Sweet Orange:

- Repels fleas, with the calming effect of the nerves, and deodorizer.

Valerian:

- Good for treating dog anxiety such as from noise and separation.

Not all essential oils are safe for use especially for dogs; hence, you need to avoid them. Here are some of those essentials oils, even in their diluted state that are still not quite safe for use on dogs.

Unsafe Oil Essentials for Dogs

Horseradish/ Mustard/ Tansy:
- May cause severe skin irritation.

Pennyroyal:
- This oil is effective in repelling fleas but is highly toxic and harmful to the kidneys and the whole nervous system.
- It is also known as an abortifacient, so avoid using it on your dogs.

Rue:
- A bad photosensitizer.

Wormwood:
- Both the herb and the essential oil derived from it are toxic for pets and must be avoided.

- Though there are suggestions that wormwood oil is good for treating worms, it is better to avoid as there had been some reports of renal failure in humans due to wormwood essence.
- It is also a common fact that wormwood causes seizures, and possesses a high degree of dermal and oral toxicity.

Anise/ Camphor / Hyssop/ Juniper / White Thyme/ Yarrow:

- Because of uterine stimulation or possible toxicity, avoid using these oils on dogs, especially on pregnant dogs.
- The oil of Juniper berry is perfectly safe, but the Juniper wood oil is toxic to the kidneys.

Birch Wintergreen:

- Some aromatherapy formulae found on websites suggest using the oils birch and wintergreen for joint pains caused by arthritis. However, dermal use of these two oils has been proven to be toxic as they contain high levels of methyl salicylate.
- Ingestion can cause severe poisoning and death.

Cassia Clover leaf and bud:
- These oils can cause dermal irritation and possible toxicity to both people and pets.

THE BASICS OF ESSENTIAL OILS FOR DOGS

Before buying or committing to any essential oil brand for your dog, here are some basic points that you should know. Also, bear in mind that every animal is different hence, be observant on how your dog responds to the various kinds of oils. Common sense and good judgment help a lot as you venture out and try different methods.

Choosing Essential Oils for Your Dog

How to Purchase Essential Oils

For starters, remember that you need to find pure and therapeutic-grade essential oils for your canine buddy. There may be a lot of markets and brands out there to buy or to try. Also, you may be confused when you find that some oils of the same kind may have a great difference on their price tags. However, the guideline outlined below should be able to help you in choosing high-quality essential oils for your dog.

- Choose essential oils in violet, dark blue, amber or cobalt-colored glass bottles as dark-colored glasses to protect the oils from degrading ultraviolet radiation, helping to preserve the potency of the essential oils.

- Choose the ones bearing important information about the oils. The information can be provided via the store's brochure, website or the product's printed label. Take note of the following information:

- ❖ Common name of the essential oil (like Lavender, Basil, Cardamom, Frankincense, Ginger, ... etc.)
- ❖ Scientific name of the oil (like Lavandula angustifolia, Ocimum basilicum, Elettaria cardamom, Boswellia rivae, Zingiber Officinalis... etc.)

- ❖ Information about the procedure on how the oil was extracted
- ❖ The country of origin of the essential oil
- ❖ How the essential oil was cultivated (like wild-grown, organic farmed, conventionally grown... etc.)
- ❖ The label "100% pure essential oil."

Now, if you want to test how "pure" the essential oil you purchased, just put one drop of it on a small piece of construction paper or white printer paper. If the oil evaporates quickly and leaves no trace on the paper, then it is truly pure. On the other hand, if you see a trace left on the paper then the oil is most likely to be adulterated or diluted. However, there are certain essential oils that are exempted from this test and such are the absolutes, myrrh, vetiver, sandalwood, German chamomile and patchouli.

- Don't choose essential oils that are unreasonably cheap for they are usually adulterated or diluted.

Note that essential oils are generally expensive and should be rightfully so. Why? Know that huge amounts of plants are harvested to be able to produce essential oils. For example, a hundred pounds of lavender plant material is equivalent to a mere pound of its essential oil. Or in the case of extracting essential oil from Bulgarian roses, one pound is equivalent to 4,000 pounds of plant material.

Just in case, remember that chamomile, rose, jasmine, lemon balm and helichrysum should always be costly.

- It is wiser for you to avoid purchasing essential oils at health food stores or supermarkets. They may be cheaper in these markets but they are more likely to be of lower quality.

How to Properly Store Essential Oils

Although essential oils do not go stale or change odor, they do oxidize, deteriorate and can lose their therapeutic properties over time. Therefore, it is important that you know how to store them properly to avoid this.

Oils like citrus oils oxidize and lose their aroma and healing properties in 6 months but not all essential oils lose or diminish their aromatic quality in the long run. Essential oils of patchouli and sandalwood have their aroma mature with age.

However, according to Robert Tisserand, one of the world's experts in aromatherapy, essential oils oxidize and therefore lose their therapeutic value in time. This is why all essential oils benefit from proper handling and storage.

Store your essential oils in amber or cobalt blue bottles. This is to protect your essential oils from deterioration and losing their aromatic as well as therapeutic value. Dark glasses help keep out sunlight which is the leading cause of deterioration. Though clear glass can't harm your essential oils, they don't protect your oils from the damaging sunlight. The same reason why beer is packed in a dark bottle to protect its content from sunlight exposure.

As much as possible, avoid purchasing or storing pure essential oils in plastic bottles as essential oils gradually "chew" on the plastic. Sometimes vendors are using lined aluminum bottles in packaging essential oils. Aluminum is acceptable if the interior of the bottles is lined to prevent direct contact with the material which could cause some chemical reaction. It is also important that you store your essential oils in cool, dark places.

Do not purchase essential oils that are stored in bottles with a rubber dropper. Rubber droppers must be kept away from essential oils as it can be turned into something gum-like and therefore ruin the essential oil.

Instead of the rubber dropper, pack them in bottles that contain an orifice reducer. The orifice reducer can act as a built-in dropper but is made of a different material than what a rubber dropper is made of. Orifice reducers are made of materials that can withstand exposure even when it comes in contact with essential oils. The orifice reducer is a handy dispensing device. You can dispense the oil drop by drop by simply tipping the bottle.

Usually, a vendor, especially a wholesaler does not necessarily provide orifice reducers to their buyers but, if you need one, it is best to inquire what type of packaging they have for their bottles of essential oils.

Overall, it is recommended that essential oils must be stored in a refrigerated environment if possible. If not, store them in a cool location and avoid keeping your essential oils in places that are prone to temperature changes.

How to Get Your Dod To Enjoy Essential Oils

Because of the strong smell of most essential oils, your dog won't like them very much. So as not to deter your dog from taking essential oils, try applying the following steps.

- Try to go slow. Start with a little dose and if your pet reacts vehemently, don't force it on them. Instead, find ways to give it to your dog in other forms.

- Watch out for your dog's reaction. Like humans, animals have their own preference for scents and they react based on how they feel towards the smell. Try changing your essential oil based on how your dog likes or dislikes. Be sure to take note of his responses so you may tell your holistic veterinarian later.

- Skin sensitivity is not uncommon among dogs. Notice if your dog paws or starts scratching in the area where an essence has been dropped as this is an indication that your dog may not like the scent at all. In this situation, you may apply carrier oil, an organic jojoba oil or coconut oil to the place where he scratches. This will help the oil to be absorbed quickly and therefore lose its smell.

• Start with the diffusion method. Prepare a diffuser and fill it up with water and 8-10 drops of the essential oil. Observe the reaction of your pet. Does he move nearer to the diffuser, or sit around? It could be that your pet will relocate to another area. There are some pets that truly enjoy diffuse essential oils in their homes.

• In the absence of a diffuser, you can instead place a couple of drops of the essential oil to your chest or wrist. Allow your pet to sniff it and get accustomed to the new smell.

• Petting therapy is the next move you can make. Get a drop of the essential oil in your palm and rub your hands to scatter the scent. Gently pat your dog on top of his shoulder blades. But don't forget to dilute your essential oil before doing this. You may dilute the essential oil with coconut or jojoba oil.

To dilute, add 5 drops of the essential oil

to a teaspoon of raw organic jojoba/coconut oil. This is a good ratio for a start. Remember that you can always add more, so just go slowly. Petting therapy along with diffusion method is a great way of enjoying essential oils with your pet.

Remember to leave a review on Amazon if you have found this book helpful.

7 Best Essential Oil Starters for Your Dog

There are many kinds of essential oils to choose from out there in the market. As a kick-start, you can try these seven most popular essential oils that are certifiably dog-friendly. Be sure to seek advice from a qualified aromatherapist or your veterinarian for proper diluting methods of these essential oils.

#1 - Lavender Essential Oil

This essential oil goes right on top of the list of most aromatherapists due to its versatile qualities. Aside from that, it is very safe for topical use. It can relieve the itch, prevent scarring and fight bacteria which are frequent on dogs. Moreover, lavender essential oil has a calming effect; thus, it can be topically applied when your dog feels anxiety and stress. For this, you can consult our calming recipe on Chapter 6.

#2 - *German Chamomile Essential Oil*

Just like lavender, German chamomile essential oil is mild and gentle on your dog's skin. It can be used when your furry pal suffers from skin inflammations, allergic reactions, burns and stings.

#3 - *Peppermint Essential Oil*

Peppermint essential oil is popularly known to be antispasmodic and can also help stimulate blood circulation that benefits your dog's skin and fur. It can also repel insects, eliminate bad breath and treat arthritis and car sickness (or motion sickness).

#4 - *Cardamom Essential Oil*

Known as a natural diuretic with antibacterial benefits, cardamom essential oil can also treat your dog's cough, soothe his nausea and normalize his appetite when he is eating less.

#5- *Niaouli Essential Oil*

A powerful healing agent, niaouli essential oil is the best alternative to tea-tree oil. Compared to the tea-tree essential oil, niaouli is much gentler hence, it is less likely to irritate your dog's skin. Aside from those, the essential oil is also antibacterial and antihistaminic.

#6 - *Frankincense Essential Oil*

Frankincense essential oil helps increase the blood supply to the brain and reduce ulcers. This kind of essential oil, in some cases, has shown to boost the immune system which is helpful in some cases of cancer.

#7 - *Helichrysum Essential Oil*

This essential oil has anti-bacterial properties as well as healing properties that reduce bleeding, tissue regeneration and inflammation. Caution, though, your dog may be averse to its smell since it is akin to the smell of a "squashed bug."

Do's and Don'ts to Remember

You are here reading this book about essential oils for dogs for a reason, right? And the reason is all about their well-being. Naturally, as pet parents, all we want is the best for our dogs. Thus, it is important to know the simple dos and don'ts in dealing with essential oils and your dogs.

• Do not use essential oils in areas near your dog's nose, mouth, eyes or genitals.

• Do not ignore your dog's reactions. He cannot directly tell you what is or what is not working on him. Thus, what you need is to closely observe his reactions. Watch out for whining, excessive scratching, sniffing and anxiety issues.

• Do not use any kind of essential oils on medium-large breed puppies under 8 weeks of age.

• Do not use the same dose of essential oils for the older, frail, sick and pregnant dogs as their healthy counterparts. Remember that they need special considerations. Just to make sure, first consult with an aromatherapist or your vet.

• Do not use the same dose of essential oils for the smaller breeds as you do for the bigger breeds. Always bear in mind that size matters.

- Do dilute oils with a diluting agent such as jojoba oil, olive oil or sweet almond oil. Dilute 80-90 percent before application. For instance, you can dilute 1 drop of essential oil with 4-5 drops of the diluting agent.

- Do introduce essential oils to your dog gradually. Do not force them to take it.

HOW TO SAFELY USE ESSENTIAL OILS FOR YOUR DOG

Since essential oils can benefit humans, in the same way, they can benefit dogs. It is still important to know that some essential oils that can be soothing and provide relief for your senses may not produce the same effect for your dogs and can, in fact, be dangerous to them. In the same way that chocolate is delicious to us and potentially deadly to dogs, certain essential oils don't affect the species the same way.

Essential oils contain active biological compounds that are quite powerful and can be useful to medical care. However, it is important that only people who are knowledgeable in essential oils are the ones to administer it, because essential oils can cause undesirable and sometimes dangerous side effects. Plants use their own manufacturer oils for many reasons and one is for security and protection. When plants are in danger of being consumed by predators, they automatically release compounds that neutralize or repel pests and pathogens. This way they are protected from them even when they can't move or get away. We can use these qualities for our benefit, but must be careful to not cause irritation through over-exposure.

Essential oils are taken in through inhalation, ingestion or contact with the skin. They are rapidly absorbed into the bloodstream and distributed to other parts of the body or tissues. Like all compounds, some chemicals have biological relations for specific tissues and only people who are trained in the use of essential oils can, therefore, use this property to choose oils that target specific tissues. Holistic veterinarians and aroma-therapists can be invaluable aids in choosing the correct oils and delivery methods depending on the problem that needs to be resolved.

Because compounds present in essential oils are very powerful, a very small amount of it can induce powerful biological reactions in every system of the body. An example is lavender oil, which has a powerful effect on the brain and creates a calming sensation. Just a small dosage of lavender oil can be used to calm your dog when he is under emotional strain or anxiety. At the same time though, too large of a dose, or a dose in too strong of a concentration can cause skin irritation. For reasons like this, it is important that essential oils be used and applied by someone with the knowledge necessary to do so safely.

Applying Essential Oils to Dogs

There are three ways to apply essential oils to your dog. In some cases, it will be easy to know which application is most appropriate. For instance, a remedy for wet dog smell will obviously be applied to the fur. It isn't always so simple though. In many instances it will be better to diffuse the oil into the air, rub it into the skin instead of fur or apply to other areas of the dog's body. Be sure to read instructions attached to the recipes thoroughly and follow them to the letter. Also keep an eye on your animal. You know best how they normally act and react to medicines. If any undesirable reaction occurs, you'll be the first to know if you just keep a close watch.

In some cases a dog will react to the unfamiliar smell of essential oils with resistance. While usually (if the correct recipes and steps are followed), the animal will quickly become used to the smell and welcome treatment, if your dog shows great or prolonged resistance, be sure to respect it. It's possible that the solution needs to be further diluted or adjusted to contain less of a certain ingredient. If your dog is strongly reluctant, wait a while and try other carrier methods, concentrations, ratios or applications. Be patient! It is worth it to let your dog come to the treatment willingly and avoid the "veterinarian jitters" that we so commonly see.

Topical Application

This is the best method of applying essential oils to your dog. They can get the most benefit from the essential oils when it is directly applied to areas of great concern.

The oil can easily penetrate through the skin, be absorbed by the tiny capillaries and travel quickly enough as soon as it reaches the bloodstream. Not only is this an efficient delivery system but, many pets enjoy the extra physical contact that it provides. Some dogs will run happily to receive their treatment, as though it's a "doggy massage." Thinking of it this way can ease the tension of caring for a sick animal and make it more pleasant for you too.

Through this method, you apply the essential oil to the body by massaging it directly or via sprites, sprays or by adding them to your dog's shampoo and conditioner. You can also mix them with salves, cream or ointments. Take note when mixing oils into pre-made solutions such as shampoos, soaps or lotions. Many of them already contain essences, frequently as a fragrance agent and you will need to keep that in mind when formulating your remedy. For example, if a natural fragrance is mentioned on the ingredient list and the shampoo smells strongly of lavender, you may need to dial back the lavender in the mixture in order to keep it in balance.

Before doing this method, remember to dilute the essential oil in carrier oils such as vegetable oils including olive oil, jojoba oil, sweet almond and many others before using. Some oils, such as cinnamon, lavender and peppermint are quite irritating in strong concentrations, so do make use of carrier oils when blending your essential oils for a more mild solution.

You can apply the essential oils to the spine, toes or pads of the dog or even to his ears. You may also spray into his coat or fur or directly to the affected areas on his body. However, remember to avoid the eyes, nose as well as the anal and the genital areas of the dog. These areas have mucus membranes which are much more sensitive than the skin. Not only may they become irritated, they may also absorb much more of the chemical compounds in your remedy than you intended. It is important to remember that your dog may lick oils or salves off of their skin and fur, especially if the feeling of it is unpleasant to them. Fully massaging the treatment into the skin or brushing it through the fur can reduce this greatly. If your dog tends to be sensitive to lotions and salves, keeping them on areas unreachable for licking or biting when possible may help. As a last resort, a cone collar may be necessary to keep an oil that isn't meant for ingestion out of the stomach.

Diffusion and Inhalation

Smell is an important function for animals, particularly for dogs. It is one of the primary ways that they experience the world and gather information about their surroundings. As soon as the nose catches up on the scent, it sends a message to the base of the brain which in turn, sends signals to other parts of the body. Emotions are directly influenced by what your dog smells. Good smells can send your dog to relax and remain calm, but the bad smell can irritate or repel him.

Dogs have a special kind of smelling system, much more sensitive than ours. Their sense of smell can reach farther than what we can in terms of distance. Through their unique ability to smell, our dogs can gather complex information from their surroundings and use this information to calculate their instincts and responses. It is because of their hypersensitivity to scent that we must make sure that we don't give them an overdose of these oils.

Diffusion and inhalation also work by dispersing tiny particles of essential oils throughout the air. There, once they cross the mucus membrane in the sinuses, they go to work not just in the brain but, in the sinuses themselves. You may have experienced this effect if you ever used mentholated cream to relieve a stuffy nose. The tissues of the nose and sinus are very sensitive even in people and more so in dogs. For this reason you must be careful not to expose your dog to diffused oils for too long or at too high concentrations.

The diffusion and inhalation method of aromatherapy uses a diffuser to bring oil vapor to be inhaled by your dog. Just leave the diffuser for about 30-40 minutes so he can inhale and absorb the oil vapor. By repeating the process twice daily within a week, you will soon see the results. However, never use essential oils for long unless to treat serious medical conditions like cancer. In this case, it must be administered under the guidance of a veterinary.

Another method of diffusion and inhalation is making a spritz. This is done by diluting the essential oil with alcohol and water, rather than carrier oils. Because alcohol is a potential irritant, care must be taken to avoid too much contact with the skin. However, especially in anxiety reducing or calming blends, spraying them into the air or a favorite piece of furniture can be very effective.

Oral Application

The oral application is the most sensitive procedure and must be done under the supervision of a holistic veterinarian. As essential oils are highly concentrated and have proven to be potent, extreme care must be taken to avoid administering an over dosage. Besides, you need to be sure what essential oils are suitable to a certain medical condition so as not to harm your dog. Some essential oils are extremely toxic, even in small amounts (a drop or less!) so only use this ingestion method if you are well trained and under the supervision of a vet.

Even if you are knowledgeable, make sure that the essence you will be using for your dog is of high quality. Remember that essential oils are most often blended. It is of the highest importance to have a source for oils that you trust. A high-quality manufacturer will ensure that you know where your oils are from, what the concentrations of essential and carrier oils are, and that your product is free from contamination. Always read labels carefully for this information. For this, you need to be sure of the kind of essential oils that were used in the mixture to avoid accidental ingestions.

Be sure to use only a drop of the essence when administering it to your dog and never force it on your pet if he shows signs of being against it. Animals are sensitive to smell, so they can easily tell what's going on. These instincts are natural in dogs and are one of the ways they protect themselves from dangerous chemicals. One way to get your animal used to the smell of essential oils is to wear the mixture on yourself for a while and interact with them. This allows them to become accustomed to the scent in a friendly and non-threatening way. This is particularly helpful because it will allow you to understand your dog's reaction properly. If it is just a bit of discomfort because the smell is new and surprising, getting used to it on you will alleviate that. If your dog still is resistant, it may be because the oil is not right for them. Trust your dog when it comes to herbs and oils. Sometimes, you can even see your dog nibbling on some kind of herbs or grasses when they are sick or with indigestion. They are natural herbalists!

For home remedies, especially when you are just starting on your journey of animal aromatherapy, just use the first two methods and refrain from applying the third one. This is one way of showing that you can be your dog's loyal best friend.

PRECAUTION AND SAFETY IN USING ESSENTIAL OILS

Cautions

While oils are used in mental activity and healing, they are potent and can, therefore, have adverse effects on your dogs. Extreme care and caution is therefore recommended when applying essential oils to your pet in any form.

Some preparations have a long history of being helpful, such as using lavender or calendula for calming aromatherapy. Other formulations have recently come on to the scene with the rise in popularity of natural treatments. These remedies should be treated cautiously, because there isn't enough information available to ensure the safety of the treatments.

Problems with essential oils lie in the fact that they may contain contaminants or adulterants. If these are present in them, more serious issues are likely to arise. To avoid this, use only essential oils from reputable companies and make sure you verify the quality of oils before using them. It is equally important to know the concentration of essential oils. With many oils, what can be helpful in limited amounts becomes irritating or even toxic in larger amounts. It is impossible to overstate the importance of knowing where your oils are from and making sure they are open and accurate about the consistency and quality.

Because dogs have highly sensitive sense of smell, always dilute your oils and make sure that you provide an escape route for your dog to have the freedom to refuse treatment, especially when diffusing your oils. One drop of the essence diluted in 50 drops of carrier oil such as grape seed is sufficient enough for use.

Since dogs metabolize and react differently to essential oils, it is always important to explore on the species-specific difference before utilizing them, especially for ingestion. I don't recommend anyone other than a professional to administrate essential oils orally. While caution is very important, there are many safe and effective methods of treating common ailments with essential oils. With proper care, these remedies are highly effective and provide comfort and relief. Additionally, many pet owners feel better giving their animals a natural treatment instead of an artificial chemical based solution.

For instance, lavender oil is highly useful, but since it does not contain any antioxidant compounds, there is every possibility that it will oxidize as it is stored. These oxidized alcohols can, therefore, aggravate your dog's condition and may even lead to allergic reactions. Maintaining your supply of oils and storing them properly is key to preventing this. Protect them from light, heat and exposure to air. Keep a close watch on the expiration dates as well.

Some essential oils can even cause kidney and liver toxicity in more sensitive breeds. To reduce the chances of sensitivity and organ toxicity, we generally use oil for no more than two weeks and then provide a rest period. Under certain circumstances — like in the treatment of cancer — we will use oils for longer periods, but this is something best left to those trained in the use of oils."

Typical Safety Precautions When Using Essential Oils on Canines

- Use essential oils that are safe and 100 percent pure on dogs and humans.
- Be sure to dilute essential oils before using on dogs. For a rough guide, add 5-6 drops of essential oil to 1 ounce or 30 ml. of carrier base oil. For 8 ounces or 240 ml. of shampoo, use 20-25 drops of essential oils.

- Use smaller amounts of diluted oil on smaller dogs, puppies and aged dogs whose health is compromised. If you are not sure if your dog's current condition can take essential oils, then start off with hydrosols.
- Never use essential oils on dogs with epilepsy or who are prone to seizure attacks. Some oils such as rosemary can trigger seizures even in humans.
- Avoid applying essential oils around the eyes, or close to the nose, anal or genital organs. These areas contain easily irritated membranes and can be susceptible to increased chemical absorption.
- Do not fail to check with a holistic veterinarian before using any essential oils on pregnant dogs. Essential oils like peppermint, eucalyptus, tea tree and rosemary must be avoided especially when your dog is pregnant.

- Some oils are not suitable for use on dogs ever, in any quantity. Phenols, such as those in Oregano and Thyme oils are not indicated for use on canines. Pennyroyal and Wormwood oils should never be used. Be sure to only use recipes that you trust, from sources that are educated in aromatherapy and holistic veterinarian practice.
- If your animal has a history of sensitive skin, be sure to patch test any topical treatment on a small area of skin before applying fully. The skin is a complicated organ and it can be hard to predict its reaction. A patch test is the safest way to prevent a large and possibly painful amount of irritation.
- Some oils can increase sensitivity to sunlight. Citrus oils, in particular, are known for this. On short-haired breeds especially, it is very important to make sure your dog's skin is not exposed to these oils and sunlight at the same time.

Doing so can increase the risk of sunburn, possibly to a large degree. Ears are a particular area of concern, because in many breeds they tend to be sunlight sensitive to begin with.

- Never assume that an oil that is safe in one application is safe in another. Some oils are therapeutic when applied topically but useless or, even worse, toxic if taken internally. This is why it is important to follow recipe and application instructions very carefully. Not only that, but make sure the source of your recipe is a trusted and educated source.

- Always make sure your supply of essential oils, carrier oils and mixtures made with them are stored properly. Above all: they must be stored out of the reach of your animals. Some oils can smell quite tasty to dogs, but if they are ingested in any but the smallest quantities they are toxic. Even a neutral oil like vegetable oil will cause digestive troubles if eaten in large amounts. Treat these ingredients and remedies as you would any other medicine by making sure there is no way your dog can access them. If you ever suspect that your dog has obtained access to them, monitor them very closely for symptoms and call your veterinarian.

- Tea Tree oil is a common home remedy for bacterial issues. However, it can be too strong for dogs, especially small ones. If you do decide to use it, be cautious at first, always do a patch test and limit the duration of exposure. Also consider that you may be able to swap Sweet Marjoram oil for it and still achieve the desired effect.

- "Hot spots" like at the joint of the legs or neck may be more sensitive to topical applications than the spine or sides would be. On animals with a lot of fur or skin, keep in mind that where the skin meets skin or stays much warmer, it can intensify the effect of the oil. If it is necessary to apply remedies to these areas, keep in mind that it may be advisable to dilute the mixture to account for this. A patch test is helpful in this instance as well.

- When using a diffuser to disperse essential oils in your home there are a few precautions that will make it safer. First, turn diffusers off when you aren't at home. Dogs are more sensitive to smells than we are, so without being able to see and monitor your pet, there is no way to know if the scent has become too strong. Secondly, keep your diffuser clean. If it becomes contaminated with dust, mold or other particulate matter, those will be diffused through your home as well. This can cause all sorts of irritation and problems and is very easy to avoid.
- Consider carrier oils carefully.

Depending on your dog's skin and where the mixture is being applied, you may see a range of reactions. With a patch test, for instance, you may see dryness or slight irritation. Sometimes this is not due to the essential oil at all, but to the carrier oil. Oils like Avocado or Coconut may simply be too heavy for your animal's particular skin and fur needs. Conversely, mildly astringent oils like Mint or Rosemary may cause irritation when blended with a very lightweight oil like Apricot Seed, but could be perfect when carried in something richer. If skin sensitivity is a concern, patch test all carrier oils on their own so you can see how your dog reacts before mixing other essential oils in.

ESSENTIAL OIL RECIPES

From insect predicaments, itch problems to stress and anxiety issues, these essential oil recipes can help you and your buddy eradicate them all.

Tick Repellent

This Rose Geranium Essential Oil recipe serves as an effective natural tick repellent that can be used by both you and your dog.

What You Need:

- Rose Geranium essential oil, 40 drops
- Witch Hazel (or Vodka), 1 tablespoon
- Distilled water, ⅓ cup
- A glass sprays bottle

All you have to do is to mix the witch hazel (or vodka if you prefer) with the rose geranium essential oil in your glass spray bottle.

Subsequently, pour in the distilled water and shake. You can then apply the spray onto your dog to keep it tick free. For storage, keep the bottle in a cool place

Flea Repellent (Flea Collar)

Make your dog flea-free with your do-it-yourself flea repellent collar. The procedure is so simple and easy that you won't even break a sweat.

What You Need:

- Cinnamon essential oil, 2 drops*
- Almond oil, 2 tbsp.
- A standard dog collar

(*Note: You can use other flea-repelling essential oils like rosemary, peppermint, cedarwood, and clove. If you want to combine oils like rosemary and peppermint, use 1 drop of rosemary and 1 drop of peppermint.)

All you need is to blend all the ingredients and apply them onto the collar. Make sure that it dries off completely before putting the collar on your pet.

Mosquito Repellent

While this recipe can be used as a mosquito repellent, it can also ward off other insects from pestering your canine best friend.

What You Need:

- Witch hazel, 14 oz.
- Lavender essential oil, 12 drops
- Lemongrass essential oil, 15 drops
- Citronella essential oil, 15 drops

Mix all the ingredients inside a glass spray bottle and shake well. You can apply the spray on your dog's collar. Alternatively, you can rub a few drops on your palms and apply the oil to your dog's coat and skin. Concentrate on areas like the neck, front legs, base of the tail and the hind legs.

Insect Repellent

Do you want pesky insects to stay away from your beloved dog? This witch hazel and essential oil blend will help you and your dog. What You Need:

- Rosemary essential oil, 10 drops
- Clove* (or Eucalyptus) essential oil, 10 drops
- Citrus essential oil (like Lemon, Grapefruit or Orange), 10 drops
- Witch hazel
- Distilled water
- A spray bottle, 8 oz.

What you need to do first is to fill your spray bottle with water but be sure not to fill all the way through. Add the witch hazel just enough to fill the balance of the spray bottle. After that, put the essential oils and shake the bottle. You can then spritz your dog with the blend to protect him from pesky insects.

(*Note: Clove essential oil is uterine stimulant. Do not use it if your dog is pregnant. Instead, use eucalyptus essential oil as a substitute.)

Now, if by any reason you want an alternative to the recipe above, here's another one for you to try:

What You Need:

- Lavender essential oil, 4 drops
- Niaouli essential oil, 4 drops
- Distilled water, 1 cup
- A spray bottle

Put the distilled water into your spray bottle and add the essential oils. Shake well before spraying the blend onto your dog's coat. Be careful to avoid spritzing some on his eyes, nose, ear, genitals and mouth. The scent of the essential oils should ward off the insects.

Now, here's another simple recipe that consists only of two ingredients:

- Rosemary essential oil, 8 drops
- Distilled water, 1 cup
- A spray bottle

Just mix the two ingredients together in the spray bottle and shake well. Spray some on your dog's coat, avoiding the critical areas such as the eyes, nose, mouth, ears and genitals. It is also important not to soak your dog's fur with too much spraying.

Itch Relief

Oftentimes, dogs suffer from dry and itchy skin called "hot spots." While the essential oil recipe we mention here can soothe the itch, serious skin irritation should always be consulted to your vet.

What You Need:

- Coconut oil, 2 oz.
- Lavender essential oil, 2 drops
- Roman chamomile essential oil, 1-2 drops
- A glass bottle

What you need to do is to incorporate the lavender and roman chamomile oils with the two ounces of coconut oil into a glass bottle. Shake the bottle very well and—voila!—it is then ready to use.

Before applying the essential oil blend, clip or trim the spot and the surrounding area with clippers. This should help you get the air onto the spot, making it easier to clean and dry that area. Spray or apply a few drops of the oil five times a day.

Alternatively, you can try this lavender essential oil and coconut (or almond) base oil blend. The measurement used here can be used in one-time application only, but depending on the size of your dog and the affected areas, you may want to make more. In that case, just use the ratio herein:

What You Need:

- Lavender essential oil, 10 drops
- Coconut or almond oil as base, 2 tbsp.

Mix these two ingredients together and apply to the irritated skin in order to reduce the itch. This can also kill the bacteria and calm the nerves of your dog.

Dog Paw Ointment

Use this recipe to soothe and soften your dog's paws. Extreme weather conditions can cause damage to your dog's paw pads, causing them great discomfort. This balm will help protect and sooth in hot, dry and cold weather.

Ingredients:

2 tbsp Fractionated Coconut Oil

2 tbsp Shea butter

2 tbsp beeswax

1 teaspoon Jojoba Oil

1-2 drops Lavender Oil

1-2 drops Thieves Oil

1-2 drops Frankincense Oil

Combine Coconut Oil, Shea butter and beeswax in a small glass. Sit the glass in a pot with some water and place over low heat. Once melted and cooled, add the essential oils then transfer in a container.

Stress and Anxiety Relief

Just like human beings, dogs feel anxiety and stress. Contributing factors such as noise; fear of new places or people; and separation from their owners can induce these negative feelings. Our special blend of essential oils recipe here is perfect for calming our anxious canine buddy.

What You Need:

- Lavender essential oil, 6- 8 drops
- Valerian essential oil, 6- 8 drops
- Sweet marjoram essential oil, 3-4 drops
- Clary sages essential oil, 3-4 drops
- Base oil like jojoba oil, olive oil or sweet almond oil, 4 oz. (or 120ml)

Simply incorporate these different essential oils and your special essential oil blend is ready to use. Rub 2-3 drops on your palms and apply it on your dog's inner thighs, flanks (or what we consider as their "armpits"), outer edges of its ears, and the areas between its toes.

Alternatively, you can also use this calming

essential oil spray:

- Lavender essential oil, 5-10 drops
- Roman chamomile essential oil, 5-10 drops
- Water, 300 ml.
- A spray bottle2

Incorporate all the ingredients into the bottle and shake. Use the spray on your dog's thighs, "armpits," toe pads and thighs.

Recipe for Hyperactivity

All dogs need to be exercised daily and their need will greatly vary from one dog to the next. However, some dogs can get hyperactive even after sufficient exercise when they are overly stimulated. Use this aromatherapy recipe to calm your hyperactive dog.

Ingredients:

120ml base oil (Jojoba Oil, Sweet Almond Oil, Olive Oil, etc.)

3 drops Bergamot Oil

4 drops Sweet Marjoram

5 drops Roman Chamomile

6 drops Lavender Oil

6 drops Valerian Oil

Rub 2-3 drops of the oil blend between your palms and apply it on your dog's inner thighs, on his armpits, between his toes and on his ear tips.

Odor Control

Dealing with the bad odor of your furry pal? Try these two recipes to get rid of that smelly problem.

The first recipe is a blend of different essential oils with an all-natural shampoo. Simply blend all the ingredients together and apply as shampoo.

What You Need:

- All-natural shampoo for dogs, 8 oz. (or 240 ml.)
- Lavender essential oil, 7-8 drops
- Chamomile Roman essential oil, 4 drops
- Geranium essential oil, 4 drops
- Sweet marjoram essential oil, 3 drops

The second recipe herein can be used as a spray to eliminate the doggie smell. All you need to do is to add the following essential oils into a cup of distilled water.

What You Need:

- Lavender essential oil, 10 drops

- Peppermint essential oil, 6 drops
- Sweet orange essential oil, 6 drops
- Eucalyptus essential oil, 3 drops
- Purified water, 8 oz.
- A spray bottle

In applying, remember to cover your dog's eyes and face with your free hand. Hold the spray about 10 inches away from and directly spritz onto your pet's body except the head. You can also use this spray to sanitize and refresh your room.

If you want a much simpler essential oil spray recipe, you can try this one instead:

What You Need:

- Purification essential oil, 15 drops
- Lavender essential oil, 5 drops
- Water, 5 oz. *
- A pinch of salt

First, you need to combine the essential oils to the salt and do a gentle stirring. After these have been blended well, gradually add water. By doing this, you allow the essential oils to be distributed into the water so these won't be floating back to the top. Lightly spray your dog with this blend before he enters your house. (* Note: Double the amount of water if you are applying this recipe for dogs who weigh below 60 pounds.)

Car Sickness

Car sickness or "motion sickness" is usually one of the issues dealt with by the pet parents. Fortunately, this problem is not altogether difficult to diagnose. Signs such as nervousness, panting, salivating, whining, excessive licking... etc., point out that your dog has this problem. In some cases, your dog may even vomit, defecate or urinate inside your car.

What You Need:
- Peppermint essential oil, 10 drops
- Ginger essential oil, 14 drops
- Base oil like jojoba oil, olive oil or sweet almond oil, 4 oz. (or 120 ml)
- A glass sprays bottle

Simply blend in together all the oils into the glass spray bottle. To use, apply or spray oil blend inside the tip of your dog's ears, on its belly and "armpits." If you want, you can also apply a few drops of the oil blend to a cotton ball and put it in front of the air vent of your car in order to circulate the scent inside.

Ear Infection

It is quite common for dogs—most especially the floppy-eared kind—to develop ear infections and this may be due to a lot of factors. There is the yeast and bacteria overgrowth, growing hair, trapped foreign body into the ear canal and ear mites. While your veterinarian can certainly give you proper instructions on how to deal with this kind of dilemma, you can also help your best buddy alleviate his ear problem with this homemade essential oil.

What You Need:

- Lavender essential oil, 15 drops
- Basil essential oil, 15 drops
- Geranium essential oil, 15 drops
- Frankincense essential oil, 15 drops
- Arborvitae essential oil, 10 drops
- A glass sprays bottle, 2 oz.
- Fractionated Coconut oil, to fill bottle for up to ¾ full

Blend in all the ingredients into the spray bottle and shake well. Also, be sure to shake the bottle before using the essential oil blend. You can use this once a week to treat the infected ear (or ears) of your dog; use once a month to prevent the recurrence of the infection most especially if your dog is prone to having it.

Arthritis

Just like aging humans, aging dogs may also suffer from arthritis. Ease your dog's pain by using this essential oil blend recipe.

What You Need:

- Helichrysum (or Frankincense) essential oil, 6 drops
- Peppermint essential oil, 4 drops
- Vetiver essential oil, 3 drops
- Ginger essential oil, 2 drops
- Fractionated Coconut oil as base, ½ oz. (15 ml)
- A glass bottle

Incorporate the ingredients together into the glass bottle and shake well. Topically apply the blend to your dog's sore joints and massage. You can also pour one to two drops onto the palm of your hands, rub and massage into the tip of your dog's ears. Do not by any means drop the oil directly to his ears as it may cause burns to the inner ears.

Increasing Appetite

If you notice your dog is losing appetite due to either sickness or old age, give him this oil blend to make him excited about food again.

Ingredients:

15ml Sweet Almond Oil

2 drops Lemon Oil

2 drops Sweet Orange Oil

2 drops Bergamot Oil

2 drops Grapefruit Oil

2 drops Lime Oil

Mix all ingredients together in a dark glass bottle. Pour 2-6 drops into your hands and massage your dog in the neck and chest.

Dog Shampoo

Even the mildest shampoo for humans can be very harsh on your dog. Just in case you ran out of shampoo (or you simply want to try a more natural product than those shampoos from the supermarket) but you have the following ingredients at home, then you can try making your homemade dog shampoo. Castile soap is proven safe and mild for your dog's skin while the essential oils listed herein can help ward off insects.

What You Need:

- Rosemary essential oil, 2 drops
- Lavender essential oil, 2 drops
- Eucalyptus essential oil, 2 drops
- Peppermint essential oil, 2 drops
- Castile soap, 1 tbsp.
- Water, 350 ml.
- Bottle (for storage)
- Aloe vera, 60 ml. (optional)

Simply mix all the ingredients together in a jar before putting it into a bottle. Be sure to shake the bottle every time you use the shampoo. Castile soap doesn't lather much compared to the commercial shampoos, but it sure can make your dog's coat squeaky clean.

(* Note: Now, if you want a more "soothing" version of this shampoo, all you have to do is to replace 60 ml. of the water with 60 ml. of aloe vera.

Dog Skin Care

Dogs do age just like us and their skin—just like ours—need some loving support. The recipe we have here can produce an instant moisturizer that you and your dog can share. Yes, it can be shared by both you and your furry pal as it is mild and gentle to the skin.

What You Need:

- Lavender essential oil, 5 drops
- Roman chamomile essential oil, 5 drops
- Frankincense (or Melrose) essential oil, 2-3 drops
- Vitamin E, 3 drops
- Jojoba (or olive) oil as base, 5 oz.
- A glass dropper bottle

Mix the ingredients well together in a glass dropper bottle. Apply 2-4 drops to the skin most, especially on the extra dry areas. However, be careful if these dry areas happen to be a result of allergies. In such case, it is best to consult your vet first.

(Note: Please be reminded that this dog skin care recipe is intended for dogs who weigh 60 pounds and above. If you want to apply this to a smaller canine, just double the amount of the carrier oil to dilute the essential oils.)

Dog Aging Support

As our dog ages, he needs extra support and it does not only stop skin-deep. This essential oil blend recipe helps aging dogs feel comfortable as it supports their skeletal system.

What You Need:

- Peppermint essential oil, 3 drops
- Lavender essential oil, 3 drops
- Copaiba essential oil, 2 drops
- Balsam fir essential oil, 2 drops
- Coconut (or any carrier) oil as base, 3 tbsp.

All you need to do is to incorporate the ingredients and directly apply it as an ointment to affected areas. Alternatively, you can apply it to the pad of the foot for faster absorption into the blood stream.

(Note: This recipe is intended for 60-pound dogs. If you want to apply this recipe to smaller dogs, you need to double the amount of the base oil in order to get a larger dilution ratio.)

Energy Booster

Some pet owners have energetic dogs who they want to calm down sometimes. However, there are other pet parents who want to boost the energy levels of their dogs. The reason for the lack of energy may vary—weight problems, lack of nutrition, aging, and even depression. They should be taken care of accordingly through your vet's advice. Meanwhile, the essential oil blend recipe mentioned here should be able to help you in boosting your dog's energy level.

What You Need:

- Lavender essential oil, 6 drops
- Rosemary essential oil, 5 drops
- Peppermint essential oil, 2 drops
- Organic vegetable oil as base (enough to almost fill the bottle)
- A bottle, 10 ml.

    Just pour the essential oils into the

bottle and add the organic vegetable base oil. Shake well before using it to gently massage your dog's spine.

CONCLUSION

Essential Oils have proved to be seasoned home remedies for people and they may as well be used on human's loyal friend. However, it must come with the right knowledge to eliminate every possible danger that could arise with the wrong information, as the anatomy of a human is vastly different to a dog's.

With the right information and proper application, you can help bring down your budget in maintaining a high-maintenance friend without truly compromising your dog's health and life. In fact, essential oils have the ability to improve your dog's overall wellbeing when done correctly.

Essential Oil Recipes for Dogs

100 Simple and Easy to Follow Essential Oil Recipes for Dogs

Julie Summers

CONTENTS

	Introduction	i
1	Recipes for Odor Control	1
2	Recipes for Itch Relief & Wound Care	12
3	Recipes to Repel Fleas, Ticks and Insects	31
4	Recipes for Calming and Relaxation	43
5	Recipes for Joint & Muscle Health	59
6	Recipes for Ear, Nasal & Digestive Health	71
7	Recipes to Boost Energy & Immune System	88
8	Recipes to improve Nail & Fur Health	97
	Conclusion	109

INTRODUCTION

This book contains proven ways that essential oils are safe and effective to use in combatting common problems associated with dogs, including bad odor, dry and itchy skin, fleas, anxiety, joint pains and reduced energy. In many cases, essential oils even exhibit better therapeutic effects than other types of treatment. In fact, several studies have shown that dogs treated with essential oils gained better and faster results than those treated with alternative medicine. So if you think essential oils and aromatherapy work only for humans, think again.

Most essential oils have been found to provide a variety of therapeutic benefits—among which are anti-infectious (antibacterial, antifungal, antiviral), anxiolytic (anti-anxiety), anti-inflammatory, sedative, expectorant and immuno-stimulant. And not only humans can reap these benefits, dogs and other animals too! While some oils are believed to be toxic to dogs (such as Tea Tree Oil), there are tons of essential oils that you can use to keep your dog looking fresh, smelling good, free of fleas, healthy and energetic. Some of the essential oils that can be used safely and effectively on dogs are Cardamon, Chamomile (German & Roman), Coconut, Eucalyptus, Frankincense, Geranium, Ginger, Helichrysum, Lavender, Niaouli, Peppermint, Sweet Marjoram, Sweet Orange and Vetiver. And rest assure, all of the oil blends and recipes presented in this book include safe ingredients that aren't going to cause any harmful effects to your furry pets. After all, dogs are still a man's (and woman's) bestfriend and we surely want only the best for them.

So if you want to try using essential oils on your dogs but unsure as to which ones work best (there are so many essential oils in the market!), use this book as your guide in preparing safe and natural oil blend recipes that your dogs will also love to have.

Thanks again for downloading this book, I hope you enjoy it!

RECIPES FOR ODOR CONTROL

1 — Refreshing Shampoo

Most dog shampoos that do not contain harmful chemicals and perfumes will clean your dog's fur, but do little to nothing about their natural dog odor. This simple recipe will help remove your dog's unpleasant odors and keep him smelling clean and fresh all day.

Ingredients:

240ml all-natural dog shampoo

3 drops Sweet Marjoram

4 drops Geranium Oil

4 drops Roman Chamomile

7 drops Lavender Oil

Mix all ingredients and use the shampoo on wet fur. You will want to massage the shampoo into your dog's wet fur and let it sit for 3 – 5 minutes for the oils to do its work; make sure to cover as much of your pet's body as you can, but avoid your dog's eyes, nose, mouth and ears. Let Rinse and towel dry.

2 — Bad Odor Spray

If you need something that will get rid of bad doggy smells rather quickly then this recipe is just what you need. This recipe is a topical mixture that you can spray once a day everyday for 2 weeks. After which you will want to provide your dog a short break of a few days as dogs are highly sensitive to essential oils compared to humans. If you wish to use this spray frequently you can use hydrosol instead of essential oils.

Ingredients:

1 cup distilled water

3 drops Eucalyptus Oil

6 drops Peppermint Oil

6 drops Sweet Orange Oil

10 drops Lavender Oil

Combine all ingredients in a spray bottle and mix well. Spray the mixture on your dog's body, but avoid contact with his face, especially his eyes.

3 — Soothing Dog Shampoo

Make this dog shampoo from scratch at home and be reassured your dog is getting the best quality ingredients every time you wash him. This homemade dog shampoo is safe for dogs and will leave a lasting fresh smell. This recipe is also gentle on dog fur with lavender, aloe vera and coconut oil to condition and enrich your dog's skin and fur at the same time.

Ingredients:

4-5 oz. distilled/purified water

4-5 oz. Aloe Vera

5 drops Lavender Oil

2 tbsp Coconut Oil

2 tbsp Castile Soap

2 drops Roman Chamomile

2 drops Thieves Oil

2 drops Citronella Oil

2 drops Purification

1 drop Cedarwood Oil

Mix all ingredients and store in a pump bottle. Massage it into your dog's coat to make him feel refreshed and smelling good. Use this shampoo like any regular shampoo you can find at the pet store.

4 — Grooming Shampoo

Use this shampoo recipe on your dog to give him a refreshing look and a lovely smell. It is best used while brushing your dog, as a detangle spray or as a finishing spray.

Ingredients:

10 oz. distilled/purified water

2 oz. Aloe Vera

1 tbsp Castile Soap

2 drops Rosemary Oil

2 drops Lavender Oil

2 drops Eucalyptus Oil

2 drops Peppermint Oil

Combine all ingredients in a spray bottle and shake well. Use this shampoo to rinse your pet and make sure to avoid contact with his eyes. It is best to only spray the body while using this recipe. This mixture can be stored for up to a month if stored in a cool dry place out of direct sunlight. There is no need to use a dark colored glass for storage as once mixed with mineral/distilled water the oils within this recipe will have a considerably shorter shelf-life.

5 — Doggy Deodorizer

This has to be the easiest recipe to managing your dog's odor. This quick and simple mixture will eliminate stinky dog smell and help deodorize your home. It's best used as a quick solution to manage the odor problems during rainy days or in humid weather. You can also spray this mixture onto upholstery, however you will want to also keep the room well ventilated if used extensively around the house. The smell of bergamot oil may irritate your dog in large quantities. Make sure your dog is capable of escaping the room the spray is used in whenever they feel like it.

Ingredients:

8 oz. purified water

10-15 drops Bergamot Oil

Combine water and oil in a spray bottle and spritz it around your dog 2-3 times per week. Avoid spraying him in the face.

6 — Easy Dry Dog Shampoo Recipe

Some dogs just don't like bath time. They'll run around the house all day trying to avoid the dreaded bath. This recipe is for those special pups that can't stand getting wet. A dry shampoo is a great alternative for occasional cleaning as it gets dirt and odor out of the fur.

Ingredients:

3-6 drops Lavender or Lemon Oil

1 cup cornstarch

1 cup baking soda

Apply the mixture on your pet and massage into his skin using your hands. You will want to let the powder mixture to sit for 5 – 10 minutes. This will allow the baking powder to deodorize your dog by absorbing the dirt and oils from the fur. Then you simply brush your dog down thoroughly to get the excess dry shampoo out of your dog's fur. This is a good dog shampoo to use from time to time. However, do not use this method too often as baking soda tends to build up in the fur.

7 - Coat Refresher

This spray is wonderful for when your dog doesn't need a bath but could use a little sprucing up in the coat department. Shake the bottle well and then spray lightly all over the coat, avoiding the face. Jojoba oil promotes a shiny coat, and basil oil stimulates circulation in the skin, meaning this is not only beautifying but keeps fur healthy too. Don't be concerned about alcohol drying the fur. It's only used here to bind the oils and water, and in such a small amount it will evaporate very quickly.

Ingredients:

240 mls. Water

15 drops ethanol (vodka works for this, or perfumer's alcohol)

5 drops Jojoba Oil

5 drops Rosemary Oil

5 drops Basil Oil

Combine ingredients in a spray bottle and shake well. This spray will keep in the refrigerator for a couple of weeks.

8 - Doggy Cologne

Maybe your pup has a fancy date, or maybe they just need a little scent spruce up. This is a wonderful spray for the day before Bath Day, when a little pick-me-up is just the thing to hold you and your pet over. The scents of Pine is clean and woodsy smelling, which is especially perfect in the fall and winter months.

Ingredients:

240 mls Water

1-2 drops Pine Oil

1-2 drops Bergamot Oil

Put into a spray bottle and shake very well before application. This solution will keep in the refrigerator for a couple of weeks.

9 - Doggy cologne 2

This is another pick-me-up scent for your pup. It's got a lighter, fresher smell than the other recipe, which makes it ideal for spring and summertime. This should be applied all over the coat, avoiding the eyes and head. It will perk up the coat and add a lovely, light scent to your dog's fur.

Ingredients:

240 mls Water

4 drops Clary Sage Oil

4 drops Jojoba OIl

4 drops Lemon Oil

Mix in a spray bottle and store in the refrigerator. This mixture will keep for about two weeks.

10 - Furniture Deodorizer

Instead of spraying your furniture with chemicals to get rid of doggy smells, try this all natural furniture spray. Vinegar and baking soda make odors disappear, while essential oils disinfect and supply a much more pleasant aroma. Make sure to do a spot test on a hidden area before using all over your furniture.

Ingredients:

140 mls Water

100 mls White Vinegar

2 tbsp Baking Soda

30 mls ethanol (vodka or perfumer's alcohol)

1 drop Lavender Oil

1 drop Lemon Oil

Mix in a spray bottle and store in the refrigerator. This mixture will keep for about two weeks.

RECIPES FOR ITCH RELIEF & WOUND CARE

11 — Skin Problem Relief

This recipe will relieve itching and leaves a soothing effect. Especially good if your dog is suffering from hotspot rashes or any other form of itching related to dry flaky skin.

Ingredients:

240ml all-natural dog shampoo

5 drops Geranium Oil

6 drops Carrot Seed Oil

6 drops German Chamomile

7 drops Lavender Oil

Combine all ingredients and massage onto your dog's body during bath time. Alternatively, you can use 120ml base oil (Jojoba Oil, Sweet Almond Oil, Coconut Oil, etc.) in place of the all-natural dog shampoo. Apply the oil blend on affected areas to relieve itching. Be sure to not apply too much of the oil based version as your dog's fur will trap the oils and collect dirt.

12 — Skin & Coat Conditioner

Apply this oil blend on your dog's skin and coat to relieve dryness and itching. It also helps with dry paws, calloused elbows and under belly skin. The added vitamin E will help your dog's skin to stay healthy and supple.

Ingredients:

2 tbsp Fractionated Coconut Oil

3 drops liquid Vitamin E

3 drops Frankincense Oil

3 drops Roman Chamomile

5 drops Lavender Oil

Mix all ingredients in a bowl and store in a glass bottle. Apply on affected skin areas as needed once or twice a day

13 — Skin Soother

This simple blend helps relieve dryness and itchiness. The lavender oil will calm your dog making them less agitated about their itch. Fractionated Coconut oil is a liquid form of coconut oil, which has had a certain fatty acid extracted out of it's pure form. This extraction makes the coconut oil easily absorbed by your dog's skin and blends well with other oils.

Ingredients:

2 tbsp Fractionated Coconut Oil

10 drops Lavender Oil

Mix the oils and massage into your dog's fur. This oil blend also helps fight bacteria and calm your pet's nerves.

14 — Oil Blend Against Yeast Infection

If your dog is still scratching, he might be suffering from a yeast infection. This oil blend is effective in discouraging the growth of yeast and helps keep your dog free from further infections. The lemon oil helps regulate yeast production by helping your dog's fur and skin stay dry.

Ingredients:

8 oz. Virgin Coconut Oil

10 drops Lavender Oil

2 drops Lemon Oil

Combine the oils in a clean glass bottle and shake well to mix. Massage the oil blend into your pet's skin at least once per week to improve skin health. This mixture will last a good month or two if you place the mixture in a dark glass bottle out of direct sunlight.

15 — Oil Blend Against Skin Disease

Some dogs suffer from dermatitis, which causes itchiness and hair loss. Here's a recipe to help fight this disease. However, please seek your vet's advice before using this mixture as the cause of dermatitis can be from various reasons.

Ingredients:

120ml base oil (Sweet Almond Oil and Coconut Oil)

10 drops Lavender Oil

10 drops Bitter Orange

5 drops Oregano Oil

5 drops Marjoram

5 drops Peppermint Oil

5 drops Helichrysum

Combine the oils and mix well. Put 2-4 drops onto the palms of your hands and massage your dog's neck, chest and back twice a day.

16 — Wound Care

This oil blend helps treat minor cuts, bruises, insect bites, scrapes and other minor wounds in dogs. This blend is a natural antiseptic that keeps small open wounds clean, helping to avoid infection.

Ingredients:

120ml base oil (Jojoba Oil, Sweet Almond Oil, Olive Oil, etc.)

4 drops Helichrysum Oil

5 drops Niaouli Oil

5 drops Sweet Marjoram

10 drops Lavender Oil

Store the oil blend in a glass bottle and include it in your first aid kit for dogs. Apply the oils directly on the wound as needed.

17 - Disinfectant Spray for Healing Skin

When the skin is healing from widespread rashes, such as those caused by poison ivy or mange, there is often a time of irritation between the main affliction healing and the skin returning to normal. Scratching, biting, or licking can make healing difficult during this time, so it is useful to speed the healing process. The best way to do this is by creating a clean, germ-free environment for healing to take place. This spray will disinfect gently, while spraying it means the sensitive skin won't need to be rubbed, as that may cause discomfort.

Ingredients:

240 mls Water

5 drops Eucalyptus Oil

5 drops Lemongrass Oil

2 drops Cinnamon Oil

Shake well before spraying on the infected area. Use sparingly, for no longer than a week or two.

18 - Dry Skin

Just as people have a skin type (dry, oily, normal) so can dogs! If you notice your dog's skin looking dry in patches underneath the fur, or flaky skin especially on the least furry bits of your dog, this can help. Coconut oil is very moisturizing, and Jasmine Oil increases the skin's ability to hold on to that moisture. Massage this balm into any dry patches a couple of times a week, and it should clear right up.

Ingredients:

30 mls Extra Virgin Coconut Oil

2-3 drops Jasmine Oil

2-3 drops Rosehip Oil

2-3 drops Argan Oil

Blend together well and keep in a small jar. Because of the coconut oil base, this will remain solid at room temperature which makes it easy to apply like a balm or salve.

19 - Rash Oil

One of the most common reasons for rashes in dogs (and in people!) is contact dermatitis. This could be from contact with anything: new detergents, cleaning chemicals, or just friction. It is usually not a big deal and resolves itself, but this balm can make the process more pleasant. If the rash persists for too long though, it might be something more serious so take your dog in.

Ingredients:

30 mls Sweet Almond Oil

3 drops Roman Chamomile Oil

2 drops Neroli Oil

Pat lightly into the affected area once a day for up to a week.

20 - Promote Proper Healing of Scar Tissue

It's a sad fact of life, but sometimes dogs get hurt badly or need surgery for a myriad of reasons. A talented veterinarian will be able to minimize scarring with proper stitching technique, but you can help with that too. This isn't just a cosmetic issue; the larger and more obtrusive the scar, the more likely it is to suffer from irritation and inflammation long after it's healed.

Ingredients:

30 mls Sweet Almond Oil

1 drop Bergamot Oil

1 drop German Chamomile Oil

1 drop Helichrysum Oil

1 drop Rose Oil

1 drop Patchouli Oil

10 drops of Vitamin E Oil (optional)

Combine all ingredients thoroughly and massage into healing scars to encourage smooth and less noticeable scarring.

21 - Burn Cream

For severe burns, obviously your dog should be seen by a vet. If the burn is very mild, or if a more serious burn is in its last stages of healing, this cream can help encourage healing. Zinc and Lavender keep the area germ-free, while Aloe Juice is healing to burns. The Olive Oil will keep the area flexible and moisturized so that the skin doesn't harden during healing.

Ingredients:

30 mls Olive Oil

10 mls Melted Beeswax

10 mls Aloe Juice

1 gram Zinc Oxide

2 drops Lavender Oil

Mix thoroughly and apply once a day until the burn is healed, or for one week, whichever is soonest.

22 - Sunburn

This affliction especially affects short-haired and light-colored dogs. Boxers and their cousins are particularly in danger of sunburn. This spray will not only speed the healing process with Aloe and Chamomile, but Neroli and Rose promote healthy skin as it heals. Because it is a spray, you won't need to touch the tender area with your hands, which your pup will definitely appreciate.

Ingredients:

30 mls Aloe Juice

1-2 drops Chamomile Oil

1-2 drops Neroli Oil

1-2 drops Rose Oil

Put all ingredients in a spray bottle, shake well, and store in the refrigerator.

23 - Healing Ointment for Paws

The skin of the paws is very different to the skin underneath your pup's fur. When it is injured there can be special challenges to ensuring that healing takes place properly. This ointment will provide lots of moisturization and anti-inflammation properties to keep the ideal healing conditions present.

Ingredients:

30 mls Extra Virgin Coconut OIl

2 drops Rose Hip Oil

1-2 drops Rose Oil

1 drop Helichrysum Oil

Massage into paws as they heal from little abrasions, small cuts, or scratches.

24 - Healing Ointment for Skin Issues

As skin issues like rashes and irritation heal, the skin can remain mildly inflamed. This mixture will disinfect and reduce inflammation. Only use this for a few days at a time, as the zinc can increase irritation if used for too long. It's important to find the balance of disinfection and soothing!

Ingredients:

120 mls Water

30 mls ethanol (vodka or perfumer's alcohol)

1 gram zinc oxide

2 drops Rosemary Oil

2 drops Rosehip Oil

Mix in a spray bottle and store in the refrigerator. This mixture will keep for about two weeks.

25 - Poison Ivy

Severe cases of poison ivy should definitely be treated by a veterinarian. If your dog only has a small rash, or is on the way to healing, this ointment can reduce itching and speed the process. Chamomile is a powerful anti-inflammatory, so it takes away the itch while reducing swelling. When swelling goes down, the body's natural healing processes are able to work.

Ingredients:

30 mls Jojoba Oil or Sweet Almond Oil

2 drops Elemi Oil

2 drops Chamomile Oil

Mix thoroughly and apply to affected areas once per day for up to a week.

26 - Bruises

Arnica is a powerful oil that is known the world over for its ability to help bruising heal. In addition to arnica, Hyssop and Parsley encourage blood flow, Geranium takes inflammation down, and the act of massaging this balm in even helps by breaking up the oxidized blood that makes up a bruise.

Ingredients:

30 mls Carrier Oil such as Jojoba or Coconut Oil

3 drops Arnica Oil

2 drops Hyssop Oil

1 drop Parsley Oil

1 drop Geranium Oil

Mix all ingredients together and gently massage into affected area.

27 - Healing Dry, Cracked Skin

Sometimes the skin can become so dry it takes on a weathered, cracked appearance. Usually this is due to long exposure to water, especially salt water. If this affects your dog after a trip to the beach, or after spending time in an unusually arid climate, massage this mixture directly into the skin for several days in a row.

Ingredients:

30 mls Coconut Oil

3 drops Rose Hip Oil

3 drops Argan Oil

2 drops Neroli Oil

Mix ingredients together well and massage in to dry skin.

28 - Sensitive Skin Inflamed

For dogs with already sensitive skin, inflammation becomes a special problem. Where some of the calming oils that are normally used might help a dog with normal skin, they can prove irritating to the sensitive pet. This spray contains anti inflammatories in a simple, pure water base that is safe for sensitive skin.

Ingredients:

240 mls Water

5 drops Turmeric Oil

5 drops Frankincense Oil

Mix ingredients in a spray bottle and spray onto affected area, parting the hair if necessary. This mixture will keep in the refrigerator for about two weeks.

RECIPES TO REPEL FLEAS, TICKS & INSECTS

29 — Flea Repellant

Use this oil blend to remove fleas, as well as a repellent when your dog goes outside. This blend is best used before you discover the presence of fleas on your dog.

Ingredients:

120ml base oil (Jojoba Oil, Sweet Almond Oil, Olive Oil, etc.)

6-7 drops Peppermint Oil

4-5 drops Clary Sage

2-4 drops Lemon Oil

4 drops Citronella Oil

Mix all the oils together and drip a few drops to your dog's neck, legs, chest, back and tail. You can also apply a few drops to his bandanna or fabric based collar.

30 — Flea Spray

This blend can be used as a spray and is more versatile in use. You can happily use this blend more regularly than the blend above. The apple cider vinegar can also help with yeast problems.

Ingredients:

1 liter distilled/purified water

1 cup apple cider vinegar

2-3 drops Cedarwood Oil

2-3 drops Lavender Oil

Combine the apple cider vinegar with the essential oils and mix well. Put the mixture in a spray bottle and spray it onto your dog's body (avoid spraying near his face). You may also spray it on his bedding to keep fleas off.

31 — Flea Spray

This is another oil blend to spray on your dog to get rid of fleas naturally.

Ingredients:

8 oz. distilled/purified water

10 drops Lavender Oil

5 drops Cedarwood Oil

5 drops Eucalyptus Oil

5 drops Citronella Oil

Mix all ingredients in a spray bottle and shake well before using. Spritz on your pet regularly and store in a dark area to preserve the efficacy of the essential oils. Sunlight will damage the essential oil properties.

32 — Fleas Around the Tail

Some owners will notice that fleas tend to favor certain places on your dog. One of these places is none other than your dog's bottom. Fleas tend to congregate at the base of a dog's tail or anus area due to the smell. Use this oil blend if your dog's tail seems to be the fleas' favorite dwelling. This blend unlike the others is suitable for this sensitive area.

Ingredients:

1 tbsp Olive Oil

2 drops Lavender or Cedar Oil

Mix oils and apply it at the base of the tail to prevent fleas from harming your pet, but avoid applying it directing onto the anus area.

33 — Flea & Tick Repellant Spray

This recipe will help discourage fleas and ticks from latching onto your dog.

Ingredients:

2 tbsp Fractionated Coconut Oil

2 drops Lemongrass Oil

2 drops Cedarwood Oil

2 drops Thieves Oil

2 drops Citronella Oil

5 drops Lavender Oil

Combine all ingredients in a spray bottle and spray on your dog's coat to get rid of fleas and ticks. Avoid contact with eyes and face when spraying.

34 — Flea & Tick Collar

Apply this oil blend on your pet's collar to drive away fleas and other parasitic insects.

Ingredients:

1 cup distilled/purified water

5 drops Lavender Oil

2 drops Citronella Oil

2 drops Purification Oil

2 drops Thieves Oil

1 drop Cedarwood Oil

Combine all ingredients in a bowl. Soak your dog's cotton bandanna into the oil blend and let it dry before using. You may also add a few drops on your dog's collar to repel lice.

35 — Tick Removal

Any pet parent who has experience with ticks will know they are hard to pull off your dog. Use this oil blend to weaken ticks so you can remove them easily.

Ingredients:

2-3 drops Palo Santo

1 drop Rosemary Oil

Apply Palo Santo on the tick for easy removal. It will die and fall off typically within 15-20 minutes. Then, apply Rosemary Oil on your dog's skin, especially on the area where the tick had been. Rosemary acts as an antibacterial and helps keep parasites off your pet.

36 — Tick Repellant

If ticks are a big problem where you live, then this natural tick repellant is what you need. Use it just like a flea repellant by spraying it onto your dog's body.

Ingredients:

120ml base oil (Jojoba Oil, Sweet Almond Oil, Olive Oil, etc.)

6 drops Lemon-Eucalyptus Oil

8 drops Geranium Oil

10 drops Lavender Oil

Mix the oils and apply it to your dog's neck, chest, legs, back and tail.

37 — General Insect Repellant

If you love spending time outdoors with your dog then you'll know how spring and summer can wreak havoc for your furry pal. Insect of all kinds come out and your curious dog can't stop getting bitten by them. Use this oil blend to keep insects off your dog.

Ingredients:

2 cups distilled/purified water

8 drops Peppermint Oil

8 drops Lavender Oil

Mix water and oils in a glass spray bottle. Spritz your dog every day with the mixture, avoiding nose and eyes. You may also spray his bedding or clothes to repel insects even while he sleeps.

38 — Mosquito Repellant

Use this recipe to keep the mosquitoes away from your dog and prevent diseases caused by such insects. Dogs with short fur are the most prone to mosquito bites as they have no difficulty biting skin.

Ingredients:

8 oz. Aloe Vera juice

5 drops Rose Geranium

5 drops Lemongrass Oil

7 drops Citronella Oil

10 drops Myrrh Oil

Mix all ingredients in a spray bottle and spray it on your dog's body before going to a mosquito prone location(avoid contact with eyes). You can also apply it on beddings and around the doorway to repel insects.

39 - Relieve Bee Stings

Bee stings are a painful and annoying, but usually not dangerous event for dogs. If you can remove the stinger safely, do so, and apply a cold compress for a few minutes, then this salve. Apply the ice afterward too to keep swelling down. Swelling is a natural response, but it impedes the healing process. Chamomile and baking soda will work together as anti-inflammatories as well.

Ingredients:

30 mls Coconut Oil

1 tsp Baking Soda

3 drops Vetiver Oil

3 drops Spearmint Oil

1 drop Chamomile Oil

Mix ingredients well and dab onto the sting.

RECIPES FOR CALMING & RELAXATION

40 — Calming Mist #1

A soothing oil blend to help your dog relax. Great for situations your dog tends to feel nervous and anxious about, such as car rides, vet visits and new situations.

Ingredients:

1 cup distilled/purified water

5 drops Lavender Oil

5 drops Roman Chamomile

5 drops Rosemary Oil

Combine all ingredients in a spray bottle and spray on your dog's coat (avoid spraying on his face). You may also rub a few drops between your palms and massage it on your dog's neck, chest and back.

41 — Calming Mist #2

Some dogs struggle to stay calm in new environments or situations. This blend will help your dog relax and stay calm, by helping the areas of the brain that is overly stimulated to become less active.

Ingredients:

1 cup distilled/purified water

5 drops Lime Oil

5 drops Lavender Oil

Mix all ingredients in a spray bottle. Spray it around your dog and avoid spraying directly on his face. You can also spray it on your palms and massage your dog's neck, chest and back.

42 — Calming Oil Blend

This is a simple essential oil recipe to help with anxiety in dogs. If your dog seems to get anxious in certain situations that causes behavioral problems, such as fearful submission (hiding in a corner, body low to the ground, unable to move etc), or fearful aggression (growling, snarling or barking etc), then this blend will help your dog to overcome this emotional barrier.

Ingredients:

8 tbsp carrier oil (Fractionated Coconut oil or Sweet Almond Oil)

2 drops Ylang Ylang Oil

2 drops Clary Sage

2 drops German Chamomile

Mix the oils together. Apply 1/4 teaspoon of the blend to your palms and gently massage into your dog's body. Administer essential oils at least 4 hours before an event that will usually make your dog feel anxious (e.g. environmental changes).

43 — General Fear & Anxiety

If you find your dog doesn't favor the strong smell of Clary Sage, you can try this recipe to calm your pet down whenever he's anxious or become fearful of things.

Ingredients:

2 oz. Jojoba Oil

4-6 drops Lavender Oil

6-8 drops Petitgrain Oil

8-10 drops Neroli Oil

Rub 2-3 drops of the oil blend on your palms and massage it on your dog's toes, ears, armpits and inner thighs.

44 — Recipe for Anxiety

Use this recipe to calm your dog who has noise/separation anxiety or fear of new people, things or places. Separation anxiety is common for dogs that have gotten use to having people around them, and think this is the normal state life should be. If you find your pup having trouble adjusting to being alone, then try using this blend to help ease this adjustment period.

Ingredients:

120ml base oil (Jojoba Oil, Sweet Almond Oil, Olive Oil, etc.)

4 drops Sweet Marjoram

4 drops Clary Sage

8 drops Lavender Oil

8 drops Valerian Oil

Rub 2-3 drops of the mixture between your palms and massage it between your dog's toes, on the edge of his ears and on his armpits and inner thighs.

45 — Recipe for Hyperactivity

All dogs need to be exercised daily and their need will greatly vary from one dog to the next. However, some dogs can get hyperactive even after sufficient exercise when they are overly stimulated. Use this aromatherapy recipe to calm your hyperactive dog.

Ingredients:

120ml base oil (Jojoba Oil, Sweet Almond Oil, Olive Oil, etc.)

3 drops Bergamot Oil

4 drops Sweet Marjoram

5 drops Roman Chamomile

6 drops Lavender Oil

6 drops Valerian Oil

Rub 2-3 drops of the oil blend between your palms and apply it on your dog's inner thighs, on his armpits, between his toes and on his ear tips.

46 — Recipe for Separation Anxiety

Try this simpler oil blend if your pet experiences separation anxiety when you leave him alone at home. This blend doesn't use a base oil to dilute the essential oils so your dog may not appreciate excessive use of this blend if you plan to use this regularly.

Ingredients:

8-10 drops Sweet Orange Oil

4-6 drops Lavender Oil

4-6 drops Ylang Ylang Oil

Combine the oils and rub 2-3 drops between your palms. Massage on your dog's armpits, inner thighs, ear tips and between his toes.

47 — For Relaxation

This is a quick and easy blend to calm your anxious or over-excited dogs. The main active ingredient here is the lavender oil. This blend is more suitable for when you're at home as this is not a topical blend, or if your dog will be in an indoor area.

Ingredients:

1 cup distilled/purified water

3 drops Lavender Oil

1-2 drops Lime Oil

Mix the oils together and pour it in a diffuser. Turn the diffuser on and you will find your pets relaxing and most possibly sleeping within 30 minutes.

48 — Calming Lavender Powder

Make a calming lavender powder for your dog who has stress or anxiety issues. Incorporate baking soda, cornstarch or rice flour to this mixture to create powder. It also works great as a quick dry bath if you use baking soda for this mix.

Ingredients:

1 part Ylang Ylang Oil

2 parts Clary Sage

2 parts Bergamot Oil

3 parts Lavender Oil

Add 12-15 drops of this oil blend to every cup of baking soda and mix well. When your dog is stressed, sprinkle powder on his blanket to help him calm down.

49 - Acute nervousness

At times of extreme stress, it can be very helpful to have a special calming scent that you and your dog can always return to. The sense of smell is deeply linked to memory, not only in humans, but many experts suspect this is true for dogs as well! Calming Valerian and Rose Geranium combine with Sesame Oil, which normalizes the nervous system response, to create soothing oil.

Ingredients:

30 mls carrier oil, such as Sweet Almond Oil

2 drops Valerian Oil

2 drops Rose Geranium Oil

2 drops Sesame Oil

Try dabbing this oil on yourself during calm, peaceful playtime with your pup, and the scent will remind them that everything's okay when they get stressed.

50 - Low Energy After Illness

Frequently, even after the "corner has been turned" of an illness, the usual vim and vigor a dog usually exhibits will be absent for a few days. This spritz is energizing and disinfectant. This is important because the immune system may still be a little low during this time, and needs to be protected.

Ingredients:

240 mls Water

15 drops ethanol (either vodka or perfumers oil will do)

1-2 drops Ylang Ylang Oil

1-2 drops Lemongrass Oil

1-2 drops Tangerine Oil

Spray this around the room your dog will be spending time in during recovery.

51 - Restlessness

Especially in "teenage" dogs, the ones who are not puppies anymore, but not quite full-grown, we frequently see them have trouble settling down. This balm will settle the nervous system and allow jumpy muscles to relax while soothing the emotions as well. Massage it into the chest and between the forelegs to provide maximum calming and balancing effects.

Ingredients:

30 mls Extra Virgin Coconut Oil

10 mls Argan Oil

1-2 drops Ylang Ylang Oil

1-2 drops Bergamot Oil

1-2 drops Clary Sage Oil

Mix together thoroughly and keep in a small jar. The texture should be like a thick serum, which makes it light enough to massage in quickly.

52 - Sleep Support

If your pet has a consistently hard time getting to sleep, even when they are clearly tired, that might be something a veterinarian should look at. If the sleep troubles are only intermittent and not caused by any underlying issue though, this diffusion can help. Valerian is a time-honored sleep inducer, and St. John's Wort calms the nervous system to help your pet stay asleep.

Ingredients:

1 Cup Water

1 drop Lavender Oil

1 drop Valerian Oil

1 drop Chamomile Oil

1 drop St. John's Wort Oil

Pour into a diffuser and turn diffuser on for 45 minutes before bedtime.

53 - Fear of car rides

A little bit of simple training combines with powerful soothing oils to banish fear of car rides. Dab a little of this oil on your body and hold your dog in calm, peaceful playtimes for a week or so. Then, when it's time to get in the car, massage it into their chest and neck. The association of happy times will calm them, while Valerian works on the nervous system to settle it.

Ingredients:

30 mls Carrier Oil, such as Jojoba or Coconut Oil

4 drops Valerian Oil

2 drops Ginger Oil

Mix thoroughly and store in a small jar at room temperature.

54 - Crate Anxiety

This is another example of how training and oils can work together. Spray this mixture on a favorite blanket and incorporate it into gentle playtime. Then, an hour before it's time to get into the crate, spray a small spritz of this inside. The association will work together with Lavender to calm the nerves. Clary Sage has been shown to boost mood and increase happiness and "home" feelings in humans. Some experts think this may work for canines as well.

Ingredients:

120 mls Water

2 drops Lavender Oil

1 drop Clary Sage Oil

Mix in a spray bottle and store in the refrigerator. Shake well before using.

RECIPES FOR JOINT & MUSCLE HEALTH

55 — Sore Joint Oil Blend #1

This recipe will soothe your pet's sore joints and ease pain caused by dysplasia or arthritis. Ginger and lemon is great for inflammation of tissue and joints while lavender can help calm the area down.

Ingredients:

120ml base oil (Jojoba Oil, Sweet Almond Oil, Olive Oil, etc.)

8 drops Ginger Oil

6 drops Lavender Oil

8 drops Lemon Oil

Mix all the ingredients. Apply the mixture topically on your dog's swelling joints and massage gently. This is best used daily on the required area.

56 — Sore Joint Oil Blend #2

Another oil blend that will ease pain and swelling in joints.

Ingredients:

120ml base oil (Jojoba Oil, Sweet Almond Oil, Olive Oil, etc.)

4 drops Peppermint Oil

7 drops Valerian Oil

5 drops Ginger Oil

8 drops Helichrysum Oil

Combine all ingredients and massage the mixture on the affected areas. You may also apply 1-2 drops on the inside of your dog's ear tips for added comfort.

57 — Arthritis Relief

This oil blend provides great comfort for pets with joint pains or arthritis. Birch oil is great for muscle aches and pains, but also very effective for chronic pain such as arthritis.

Ingredients:

7 drops Rosemary Oil

8 drops Juniper Oil

12 drops Birch Oil

Mix the oils together and apply directly on painful and sore joints. Massage the affected area twice per day to soothe the pain away.

58 — Arthritis Oil Blend

This blend uses frankincense oil to actively treat arthritis. Frankincense has long been used as a cure for arthritis in India and has recently been scientifically proven for it's healing properties. However do consult your vet before use as the amount of frankincense oil used should correlate to the weight of your dog.

Ingredients:

½ oz. Fractionated Coconut Oil

6 drops Frankincense or Helichrysum Oil

4 drops Peppermint Oil

3 drops Vetiver Oil

2 drops Ginger Oil

Mix the oils and use topically to relieve sore joints and pain caused by arthritis. Rub a few drops on your palms and massage into the affected areas. You can also apply a few drops on your dog's ear tips for extra comfort.

59 — Rheumatism Oil Blend

As they age, dogs suffer from rheumatism just like humans. Prepare this blend to help you aging pal cope with the swelling of joints.

Ingredients:

7 drops Rosemary Oil

8 drops Birch Oil

8 drops Juniper Oil

Pour these oils in a 10-ml dark glass bottle and mix well. Apply 2-4 drops to your hands and massage your dog in the neck, chest and back to alleviate pain. Do this in the morning and at night before sleep.

60 — Muscle Ache Ointment

This mixture helps soothe muscle aches and pain in dogs. Some breeds that are prone to hip dysplasia will find this blend helpful in soothing the thigh muscles.

Ingredients:

1 tbsp Fractionated Coconut Oil

3 drops Lavender Oil

2-3 drops Copaiba Oil

Combine all the oils and store in a glass bottle. Whenever your dog is showing symptoms of sore muscles, rub the mixture on the affected area(s) for immediate relief.

61 — Dog Paw Ointment

Use this recipe to soothe and soften your dog's paws. Extreme weather conditions can cause damage to your dog's paw pads, causing them great discomfort. This balm will help protect and sooth in hot, dry and cold weather.

Ingredients:

2 tbsp Fractionated Coconut Oil

2 tbsp Shea butter

2 tbsp beeswax

1 teaspoon Jojoba Oil

1-2 drops Lavender Oil

1-2 drops Thieves Oil

1-2 drops Frankincense Oil

Combine Coconut Oil, Shea butter and beeswax in a small glass. Sit the glass in a pot with some water and place over low heat. Once melted and cooled, add the essential oils then transfer in a container.

62 - Muscle Soreness

This oil blend is particularly effective for sore muscles caused by large amounts of exercise or exertion. Even young, healthy dogs can be left feeling stiff after a long hike or swim, and this will help. Because the oils used are quite strong and invigorating, use this only for a day or two at a time and then stop. This should not be used on animals that are known to have issues with dry or sensitive skin.

Ingredients:

30 mls Fractionated Coconut Oil

1 drop Juniper Oil

1 drop Cyprus Oil

1 drop Eucalyptus Oil

1 drop Orange Oil

1 drop Peppermint Oil

Blend oils together well and rub vigorously into sore muscles. One application should be sufficient to soothe sore muscles.

63 - Painful Joints

Joint pain isn't always caused by arthritis or rheumatism. Sometimes during injury recovery or just from exertion, temporary joint pain is the result. This oil will soothe the pain and also encourage recovery.

Ingredients:

30 mls Carrier Oil, such as Jojoba or Coconut

2 drops Turmeric Oil

2 drops Vetiver Oil

2 drops Ginger Oil

Massage lightly into affected joints daily, for up to a week.

64 - Sore Spine

Back pain is particularly hard to bear, even for people. Our achy dogs might not be able to tell us when they have a sore back, but it's our job to know! Watch for a usually jumpy dog that seems reluctant to move around, and massage this oil directly into the skin above the spine. As always, make sure that if the symptoms persist more than a few days you get a professional opinion.

Ingredients:

30 mls Carrier Oil, such as Jojoba or Coconut Oil

1-2 drops Wintergreen Oil

1-2 drops Cypress Oil

Mix all ingredients well and store in a small jar.

65 - Ligament Pain

Both injury and age can cause the particularly gnawing pain that happens in the ligaments. The Black Pepper Oil in this blend increases circulation, while Lemongrass and Sweet Almond Oil are soothing. A few minutes of massaging this into the affected joint once a day for up to a week should ease the pain as the joint heals itself.

Ingredients:

30 mls Carrier Oil, such as Jojoba or Coconut Oil

2 drops Lemongrass Oil

2 drops Black Pepper Oil

10 drops Sweet Almond Oil

Mix all ingredients thoroughly and store in a small jar

RECIPES FOR EAR, NASAL & DIGESTIVE HEALTH

66 — Ear Infection Ointment #1

This oil recipe will help prevent and treat common ear infections among dogs. If your dog is prone to earwax building up in their ear canal then you can use this after cleaning their ears once a month.

Ingredients:

120ml base oil (Jojoba Oil, Sweet Almond Oil, Olive Oil, etc.)

5 drops Bergamot Oil

5 drops Niaouli Oil

6 drops Roman Chamomile

8 drops Lavender Oil

Combine the oils in a glass bottle and mix well. Massage the outside of your dog's ear with the oil blend and apply a few drops into his ear canal using a dropper.

67 — Ear Infection Ointment #2

Another oil recipe that will help treat ear infection and prevent it from coming back.

Ingredients:

2 tbsp Fractionated Coconut Oil

10 drops Arborvitae

15 drops Basil Oil

15 drops Frankincense Oil

15 drops Geranium Oil

15 drops Lavender Oil

Combine all ingredients in a glass bottle and shake well to mix. Use this oil blend once per week to treat ear infection or once per month to prevent recurrence of the infection.

68 — For Ear Health

This oil blend encourages healthy function in your dog's ears. Lavender oil is gentle and effective in cleaning out dirt from your dog's ears.

Ingredients:

1 tbsp Fractionated Coconut Oil

5 drops Geranium Oil

5 drops Melaleuca Oil

5 drops Lavender Oil

Mix all ingredients and store in a glass bottle. After cleaning your dog's ears with an all-natural cleaner, use a cotton bud to rub a few drops in his ears. Don't push the bud in where you cannot see it. Do this twice per day until you see improvement.

69 — For Sinus Infections

This oil blend is effective in relieving nasal congestion and allows your dog to breathe more easily. This is great for brachycephalic dog breeds who can experience breathing difficulties in hot weather.

Ingredients:

120ml Sweet Almond Oil

2 drops Niaouli Oil

4 drops Myrrh Oil

8 drops Eucalyptus Oil

Combine all ingredients in a glass bottle. You can either massage several drops into the neck and chest of your dog or apply it to his bandanna. You can also add several oil drops on his bedding to relieve nasal congestion.

70 — Tummy Ache Ointment

Use this recipe to help ease upset stomach and bring back your dog's vivacity. DiGize oil is famous for it's effectiveness to regulate the digestive system and sooth digestive pain.

Ingredients:

1 tbsp Fractionated Coconut Oil

3 drops Peppermint Oil

2-3 drops DiGize Oil

Combine the oils in a glass bottle. If you see your dog exhibiting signs of an upset tummy, rub a few drops on your dog's belly and massage gently with your hands.

71 — Flatulence Oil Blend

It may be comical to hear your dog toot, but just like humans, dogs can have painful uncomfortable gas. This oil blend can greatly help in alleviating flatulence caused by excess gas.

Ingredients:

15ml base oil (Sweet Almond Oil, Jojoba Oil, Hazelnut, etc.)

3 drops Tangerine Oil

3 drops Nutmeg Oil

3 drops Cinnamon Oil

3 drops Cardamom Seed Oil

3 drops Caraway Oil

Combine the oils and store in a dark glass bottle. Place 2 drops on your dog's food and administrate another 1-2 drops after eating.

72 — For Motion Sickness

Use this oil blend to calm the stomach of your dog if they are prone motion sickness.

Ingredients:

120ml base oil (Jojoba Oil, Sweet Almond Oil, Olive Oil, etc.)

10 drops Peppermint Oil

14 drops Ginger Oil

Apply the mixture to your dog's ear tips, belly and armpits. When travelling, add a few oil drops to a cotton ball and place it in front of your car's air vent to allow the scent to circulate.

73 - Heavy Breathing

Sometimes for what seems like no reason, our dogs' breathing becomes slightly labored and noisy. Usually it is just a little sinus trouble that can be soothed by inhaling this blend of anti-inflammatory sandalwood, eucalyptus, and peppermint diffused into the air for 30 minutes. If your dog's breathing issues persist though, make sure to take them in to the vet, as this can sometimes be a sign of bigger problems.

Ingredients:

4 drops Sandlewood Oil

2 drops Frankincense Oil

2 drops Eucalyptus Oil

1 drop Peppermint Oil

1 cup Water

Pour into your diffuser and turn on the diffuser for about 30 minutes.

74 - Digestion Trouble

Trouble digesting food can come from many sources. We frequently see this in animals who are recovering from more severe stomach ailments. Oils can encourage proper digestion simply through inhalation. When the food is being properly digested, appetite should increase and demeanor should also improve. Remember, if your dog appears to have trouble digesting for more than a few days, take them into the vet for examination.

Ingredients:

1-2 drops Ginger Oil

1-2 drops Fennel Oil

Apply these oils to a bandana and tie around your dog's neck with the oiled side facing outward, so the scents are easily inhaled and no direct skin contact is being made.

75 - Ear ache Massage Oil

This oil is not designed to treat ear infection, as some of the other recipes are. This can be used in conjunction with those just to ease pain and inflammation, and facilitate massage that can ease the pressure and discomfort that goes along with earache. Even without an infection, ear pain is not uncommon. If you see your dog rubbing its ears on the floor or other surfaces, this can help soothe that discomfort.

Ingredients:

30 mls Carrier Oil, such as Coconut Oil or Jojoba

1-2 drops Cassia Oil

1-2 drops Frankincense Oil

Mix ingredients thoroughly and massage directly on the ears.

76 - Heartburn

Yes, dogs get heartburn too! Some of the signs that your pet has heartburn or acid reflux are spitting up food, whining/howling while swallowing, and hacking. If this persists for more than a few days, the dog should be seen by a veterinarian. For a day or two at a time though, this might just do the trick. Since this is taken orally, be sure to keep the amount of oil in proportion to your dog's body size. Dogs under 30 lbs should use the smaller amount.

Ingredients:

1-2 drops Chamomile Oil

1-2 drops Marjoram Oil

Add to no more than one meal per day.

77 - Seasonal allergies

The uncomfortable stuffiness that accompanies hay fever is just as uncomfortable for our four-legged friends as it is for us. If your pet doesn't tolerate a diffuser well, this salve can be rubbed into the fur of the chest and between the forelegs, and the oils will waft through the nose and sinuses.

Ingredients:

30 mls Carrier Oil, such as Jojoba or Coconut Oil

1 drop Peppermint Oil

1 drop Juniper Oil

1 drop Rosewood Oil

Blend thoroughly and massage into your dog's chest to relieve stuffed-up sinuses.

78 - Sinus Inflammation

Signs of sinus inflammation might be things like snoring or loud breathing during the day. This could be caused by something more serious, and if it persists past a week you should take your dog into the vet to make sure everything is ok. If it's something simple like dryness in the air or sensitivity to something in their surroundings though, this diffusion will work wonders.

Ingredients:

1 cup Water

1 drop Eucalyptus Oil

1 drop Peppermint Oil

1 drop Turmeric Oil

1 drop Frankincense Oil

Pour ingredients into your diffuser and turn it on for 30 minutes. The smell can be quite strong at first, so make sure your dog has a way to leave the room if it becomes overwhelmed.

79 - Decrease Appetite

As sad as it is, sometimes our furry friends gain a little more weight than is healthy for them. If your veterinarian has prescribed a weight-loss strategy for your little buddy, this massage oil can make the process a little easier and less frustrating for you both. Massage this into the skin and fur of the chest and between the forelegs between meals to stave off appetite.

Ingredients:

30 mls Carrier Oil, such as Jojoba or Coconut Oil

2 drops Grapefruit Oil

1 drop Peppermint OIl

1 drop Fennel Oil

Mix all ingredients well and store in a small jar.

80 - Doggy Breath

As much as we love them, we can all admit that our pups' breath doesn't always smell the freshest. Persistent halitosis can be a sign of underlying problems, so if the problem lasts more than a week or so, make sure to take them in. If not, this mixture added to a treat or biscuit can help greatly. Because this is taken internally, make sure to monitor the amount very carefully.

Ingredients:

1 drop Peppermint Oil

1 drop Cassia Oil

Place mixture on a treat or biscuit once a day, for no more than 4 or 5 days.

81 - Vomiting

Obviously vomiting can be caused by some really unpleasant things, so make sure your dog gets the veterinary attention they need if they are vomiting. If the vomiting and nausea is something that just has to be waited out, this remedy can help. Just dab these oils on a bandana and tie around the dog's neck. The olfactory effects they have reduce nausea.

Ingredients:

1 drop Ginger

1 drop Cardamom

1 drop Peppermint

Tie around the neck with the oil facing out toward the room, away from the skin.

RECIPES TO BOOST ENERGY & IMMUNE SYSTEM

82 — For Energy Boost

This oil blend will boost your dog's energy and keep him energized all throughout the day.

Ingredients:

2 drops Peppermint Oil

5 drops Rosemary Oil

6 drops Lavender Oil

Pour the essential oils in a glass bottle and mix well. Massage a few drops on your dog's spine every morning to give him a good head start.

83 — Fatigue Oil Blend

Use this oil blend to revitalize your dog who is suffering from malaise and fatigue caused by an illness, old age or overactivity.

Ingredients:

15ml base oil (Sweet Almond Oil, Jojoba Oil, Hazelnut, etc.)

3 drops Ylang Ylang Oil

6 drops Tangerine Oil

7 drops Rosemary Oil

Combine oils in a glass bottle and mix well. Add 2-4 drops to your dog's food as needed. Be cautious in using Rosemary if your dog is prone to seizures.

84 — Increasing Appetite

If you notice your dog is losing appetite due to either sickness or old age, give him this oil blend to make him excited about food again.

Ingredients:

15ml Sweet Almond Oil

2 drops Lemon Oil

2 drops Sweet Orange Oil

2 drops Bergamot Oil

2 drops Grapefruit Oil

2 drops Lime Oil

Mix all ingredients together in a dark glass bottle. Pour 2-6 drops into your hands and massage your dog in the neck and chest.

85 — Immune System Oil Blend

This recipe may help improve your dog's immune system as the oils naturally have medicinal properties.

Ingredients:

1 cup distilled/purified water

5 drops Lavender Oil

5 drops Frankincense Oil

5 drops Roman Chamomile

Mix all ingredients in a bottle and spray it on your dog's body but not on his face. You may also apply a few drops of the oils on your palms and massage your dog's chest, back and neck area.

86 — Immune Support

Besides giving them a grain-free diet, add this simple oil blend to your dog's food to encourage strong immune system.

Ingredients:

1 drop Lavender Oil

1 drop Lemon Oil

1 drop Peppermint Oil

Combine the oils and mix well. Place it in a capsule to give to your dog or put it in his food for a healthier repast.

87 - Fever

Dogs' internal body temperatures naturally run higher than in people, so don't assume your dog is feverish just because they feel a little warm. If, however, your pet has been diagnosed with a fever due to some infection or other condition by a vet, this ointment can help to alleviate it. Make sure the underlying cause of the fever is being treated; this remedy is just to provide comfort and boost immunities while your dog recovers.

Ingredients:

30 mls Carrier Oil such as Jojoba or Coconut Oil

3 drops Garlic Oil

2 drops Eucalyptus Oil

1 drop Peppermint Oil

Mix ingredients well and massage into the neck and chest.

88 - Headache

Some symptoms of headache in dogs are low energy, avoiding sounds more than usual, and rubbing the head or ears on walls or other surfaces. If it's just a sporadic thing it's usually nothing to worry about, but if this happens frequently, make sure to take your dog in to make sure there no serious underlying cause. This ointment can help relieve pressure and pain while providing immune protection to prevent your pet from getting sick while its immune system may be low.

Ingredients:

30 mls Carrier Oil such as Jojoba or Coconut Oil

3 drops Spearmint Oil

2 drops Helichrysum Oil

2 drop Lavender Oil

1 drop Roman Chamomile Oil

Mix ingredients well and massage into the neck and spine.

89 - Antibacterial Spray

This is a great all-purpose spray to have in your refrigerator. It can be used as an air spray, on dog beds, or on the coat if there is concern about bacterial exposure. This is a nice first line of defense against getting sick if you've had a sick visitor, or been around other dogs who are sick. Always check sprays meant for fabrics in an inconspicuous spot before use. This also boosts the immune system to prevent infection.

Ingredients:

120 mls Witch Hazel

15 mls Baking Soda

1-2 drops Lemongrass Oil

1-2 drops Palmarosa Oil

Combine in a spray bottle and shake before using.

RECIPES FOR NAIL & FUR HEALTH

90 - Nail Health

Your dog's nails aren't just cute little fingernails for pups! They are also important tools dogs use to dig and explore the world. Because they are exposed to so many irritating and drying conditions down there on the ground, it's nice to keep them healthy with a cuticle massage after bath time. This serum is perfect for keeping a healthy pup's nails as healthy as it is.

Ingredients:

10 ml Carrier Oil, such as Sweet Almond or Jojoba

1 drop Carrot Oil

1 drop Balsam Fir Oil

Mix well in a dropper bottle, and drop one drop on each nail, massaging it in as you go.

91 - Nail Antifungal

Signs of fungus at the root of the nail can be peeling skin, flaky cuticles or a dusty appearance to the nail (even when the nails are clean). If this condition persists for more than a week or two, your dog should be seen by a vet, but this serum might be what it takes to sort it out. Lemon and Geranium oil are wonderful antifungal agents, and Coconut oil will replace moisture lost to the infection.

Ingredients:

10 mls Fractionated Coconut Oil

1 drop Lemon Oil

1 drop Geranium OIl

Mix ingredients together in a dropper bottle. Apply a drop to each nail, massaging as you go.

92 - Weak nails

There are many possible underlying causes for the nails becoming weak. Some of them can be quite serious, so if your dog suddenly develops this issue you should have them checked out. On the other hand, some dogs naturally don't have the sturdiest of nails. This serum will help strengthen them.

Ingredients:

30 mls Sweet Almond Oil

2 drops Geranium Oil

2 drops Lemon Oil

5 drops Jojoba OIl

Mix together in a dropper bottle. Apply one drop to each nail after bath time, massaging as you go.

93 - Hair Loss

Whether your dog has developed bald spots because of skin issues or injury or he's had to be shaved because of surgery, you can encourage the hair to regrow quickly and healthier than ever. Note: Make sure the underlying cause of the hair loss has been addressed. Depending on what it is, it could seriously affect the health of your pet.

Ingredients:

30 mls Grapeseed Oil

10 mls Jojoba Oil

2-3 drops Cedarwood Oil

2 drops Rosemary Oil

2 drops Lavender Oil

Mix all ingredients and massage into affected area a few times a week for up to two weeks.

94 - Hair Thinning

This differs from localized hair loss, because it's an all-over thinning of the coat. Again, make sure there is no serious underlying cause, and then you're free to use the all-natural and highly effective spray. The Cedar and Sage oil work together on the skin to encourage regrowth, and the Rosemary Oil ensures that the hair grows back healthy and strong.

Ingredients:

240 mls Water

5 drops Cedar Oil

5 drops Sage Oil

5 drops Rosemary Oil

Mix all ingredients in a spray bottle and store in the refrigerator. Spray all over the coat, avoiding the face and head, two or three times a week for up to two weeks.

95 - Seborrhea (oily skin)

Just like people, dogs can have oily, greasy skin. It isn't usually a health concern, but it can cause the fur to become lank and greasy, and oil trapped on the skin's surface can cause irritation and even pustules. This spray will help. Spray it all over the skin, parting the hair if necessary, and massage it in thoroughly. Most animals respond wonderfully to treatment once a week.

Ingredients:

100 mls Witch Hazel

2 drops Neroli Oil

2 drops Argan Oil

1 drop Lemon Oil

Mix in a spray bottle and store in the refrigerator. This mixture will keep for about two weeks.

96 - Burr Repellant

After a fun day out in the woods or fields, your dog may be happy, but he will almost definitely be covered in burrs. This oil is a great trick for preventing the long minutes of painful grooming to get them out. Simply massage this oil throughout the fur, especially on the legs and sides before a day out in the wilderness. Fewer burrs will stick, and the ones that do will come out much more easily.

Ingredients:

40 mls Fractionated Coconut Oil

4 drops Almond Oil

4 drops Sesame Oil

Combine all ingredients and massage into fur.

97 - Excessive Shedding Shampoo

Most animals shed, at least a little bit. This shampoo can reduce that amount, which is a blessing if your pet happens to shed more than usual. Swap this shampoo in for the normal one that you use every third or fourth bath. The essential oils will strengthen the hair roots and save you some grooming time.

Ingredients:

100ml distilled/purified water

100ml Jojoba oil

2 tbsp Coconut Oil

2 tbsp Castile Soap

2 drops Roman Chamomile

2 drops Neem Oil

1 drop Cedarwood Oil

Mix all ingredients thoroughly and shampoo as you normally would.

98 - Fur Detangler

Whether you have a long-haired beauty you brush frequently, or have recently adopted a tangled, messy little buddy, there are times when knots need to be worked out of the fur. This mixture of slippery oils and deodorizing Apple Cider Vinegar works wonders. Oils slide the knots apart and ACV makes sure that any trapped odors disappear right away.

Ingredients:

120 mls Water

40 mls Apple Cider Vinegar

10 drops Jojoba Oil

2 drops Rosemary Oil

1 drop Rose Hip Oil

Mix well in a spray bottle and spray on sections of hair at a time as you brush.

99 – Cracked nails

Dogs love to run and when they run on hard surfaces for a long time, your doggy pal is bound to crack a nail eventually. Damaged nails can cause discomfort or even pain in the worse situation. This recipe can be applied once everyday to help strengthen your dog's nails overtime. You'll notice them not cracking or splitting as often.

Ingredients:

10ml Grapeseed Oil

10ml Jojoba Oil

3 drops of Neem Oil

Mix the ingredients together and store in a cool dry place, out of direct sunlight. You can also add this mixture to melted beeswax to produce a waxing balm once harden.

100 – Shiny Coat

Some dogs are prone to dry flaky skin, which not only makes their coat look dull and brittle, but also causes your pal to be a itchy miserable mess. Use this recipe when you have time to really pour your attention onto your dog. The key ingredient here is oatmeal and Jojoba Oil, where both ingredients help regulate the skin's natural ability to take care of itself. The added lavender oil is added as a calming agent.

Ingredients:

Powdered Oatmeal

30ml Jojoba Oil

3 drops of Lavender Oil

Run a bath with lukewarm water and pour in powdered oatmeal until the water is sufficiently cloudy. You can buy any unsweetened oatmeal and blend it in a blender for a few minutes to get it powdered. Then add the rest of the ingredients in and massage your dog's fur and skin. You'll want your dog to soak in the bathtub for a good 10minutes before towel drying.

CONCLUSION

I hope this book was able to help you resolve all your dog's problems in a safe and effective manner. These 50 simple essential oil recipes can certainly go a long way to maintaining health and wellness of your four-legged companion!

However, these recipes still need to be administrated correctly for your dog to reap the full benefits essential oils can have. Your four legged friend is built very different to you and without the proper knowledge of how essential oils work, you may unintentionally do more harm than good.

I recommend you to fully educate yourself with the basics of essential oils before administrating any of these recipes as dogs come in many shapes and sizes with their own personal health quirks. Educating yourself with more knowledge will do wonders to how well your dog will benefit from these recipes and prevent unwanted harm.

Aromatherapy for Dogs

Julie Summers

Copyright © 2017 Julie Summers

All rights reserved.

This book is or any part of it may not be reproduced in any written, electronic, recording, or photocopying without written permission of the publisher or author having intellectual rights over the content of the book. The exception would be in the case of brief quotations embodied in the critical articles or reviews and pages where permission is specifically granted by the publisher or author.

Although every precaution has been taken to verify the accuracy of the information contained herein, the author and publisher assume no responsibility for any errors or omissions. No liability is assumed for any damage or damages that may result from the use of information contained herein.

Information contains in this book in solely for information purposes and does not intend in any way to replace professional medical and health advices rendered by practitioners in the field of veterinary medicine and you are further recommended to seek professional advice before using this material.

ISBN:
ISBN-13:

CONTENTS

1	INTRODUCTION	1
2	WHAT ARE ESSENTIAL OILS?	3
3	WHAT CAN AROMATHERAPY HEAL WITH?	10
4	SAFETY MEASURES BEFORE USING ESSENTIAL OILS WITH YOUR DOGS	22
5	IS AROMATHERAPY SUITABLE YOUR DOG?	36
6	DIFFERENT AROMATHERAPY APPLICATIONS	51
7	AROMATHERY TOOLS AND MATERIALS	61
8	3 GREAT AROMATHERAPIES FOR YOUR DOG	70

INTRODUCTION

Essential oils have previously been used for enhancement of well-being in humans but, are they safe to use on animals and pets, particularly on dogs that have been proven to be loyal companions of people?

The holistic approach to the use of essential oils for dogs is now gaining popularity among pet and dog lovers but misinformation has also taken its toll on some who were misguided in the proper ways of using essential oils on dogs. Through this eBook, we aim to correct this misinformation and provide you with a safe and easy to follow guide you can use while applying essential oils to your dog.

In this Book, you can expect a thorough understanding of essential oils on dogs including its various applications, benefits, safety precautions and uses plus, added homemade recipes which are sure to help you minimize your budget while maintaining your dog's health and well-being.

Through this guide, you can provide your pet the essential care he needs to improve his health condition, stabilize his mental and emotional state and improve his behavior.

This holistic approach to aromatherapy is geared towards enhancing the total well-being of your dog and likewise, developing a stronger bond between the two of you.

WHAT ARE ESSENTIAL OILS

An essential oil is an organic compound substance taken from the sac, glandular hair and in any other parts of the plants including leaves, roots, seeds, fruit or flowers. They are the essence of that particular plant and are responsible for the unique scent of that specific plant. An essential oil is volatile and therefore evaporates easily in addition to being diffusible.

Essential oils need to be diluted before each use as they are highly concentrated. Each essential oil carries individual properties like color, scent, healing effects and other chemical properties.

Many of these essential oils are

antibacterial, antifungal, antiviral, antioxidant and anti-inflammatory. They also affect the emotional function of the body by stimulating particular areas of the brain and can even be a sedative.

When you extract essential oils from plants through steam distillation, you can produce hydrosol, a water-based substance, which is a by-product obtained from the initial process. Hydrosol contains only a little part of the essential oil and a large part of the water-soluble parts of the plants. Unlike essential oils which are highly concentrated, hydrosol is not concentrated and can be used undiluted. You can also add essential oils for a combined effect.

For a highly sensitive dog, you can have hydrosol as an alternative option from using essential oils.

How are Essential Oil Made?

To extract a plant's essential oil, you may use the following methods:

- Steam Distillation

- Solvent Extraction
- Carbon Dioxide Extraction
- Manual Extraction

Distillation

The majority of essential oils are produced by the process of distillation. In distillation, water is heated to produce steam, which carries the most volatile substance of the scent. Then the steam is chilled in a condenser and the distilled result is collected. Normally, the essential oil is lighter and so it floats on top of the hydrosol, which is the distilled water component. Later, you will be working on separating the two compound elements.

Steam Distillation
Steam distillation uses an external source of steam, which carries the steam through the pipes into the distillation unit, sometimes at high pressure. Then the steam will pass through the aromatic material and exit into the condenser.

Hydrodistillation
The part of the plant which is used for oil extraction is fully submerged in water,

producing the "soup". When steamed, it contains the essential oil or essence. This process is the oldest method and yet the most versatile and is used in primitive countries. However, there is a risk in this method as the distiller can dry up or overheat giving the essence a burnt smell.

Hydrodistillation works best with powders like spice powders, ground wood and many other tough parts of the plants like the roots as well as other hard materials such as nuts.

Water and Steam Distillation
This method is best for distilling leafy materials but is not applicable for seeds, wood, or roots.

In this method, the leaves are placed in a steamer basket over boiling water, exposing it to the rising steam vapors.

Solvent Extraction

Some flowers used for essential oils like Jasmine and Linden blossom are too delicate to survive the process of distillation. To be able to capture their essence, the process of solvent extraction is used. The blossoms are placed in perforated trays and loaded into an extracting unit. The blossoms are then washed repeatedly using a solvent, usually hexane.

The solution dissolves all the extracted materials which include non-essence wax, highly volatile essential oil and pigments. The solution, with all these dissolvable plant materials and the solvent, is then filtered.

The filtration process is done by subjecting the whole solution to low process distillation to recover the solvent for reuse. The remaining materials that are wax-like are called the concrete and contain as much as 55% of the volatile oil.

To dilute the pure essential oils, it is again processed to remove the wax-like material. To separate the wax; it is warmed and mixed with ethanol alcohol. It is during the heating and stirring process that the concrete is broken up into small globules.

Along with the essence, some wax is also dissolved and can only be removed by freezing the solution at a very low temperature or around 30 degrees Fahrenheit. This way, the wax is separated. As a final precaution, the pure essence is now filtered and declared absolute. This extraction process actually yields three products that you can use. One is the concrete used for solid perfumes, the pure essential oil and the floral waxes which are used as additives to candles, thickening creams and lotions as an alternative to beeswax.

Carbon Dioxide Extraction

When Carbon Dioxide (CO_2) is exposed to high pressure, it changes into liquid form. Its liquid form can be chemically inactive and safe which can then be used to extract the aromatic molecules in a process akin to how the absolutes are extracted. With this process, there will be no traces of solvent residues because $CO2$ is again exposed to normal pressure and temperature. It will only revert to its gaseous form and evaporate.

Cold Pressing

Notice that when you score or zest the skin of an orange, you get to see the spray of its essential oil. In the process of cold pressing, machines are able to do just this way. They can mass-produce citrus oils by doing the same procedure—scoring the rinds and capturing the oil that comes out of them. While citrus oils can also be produced through the steam distillation process, the result seems to be of lower quality compared to the ones produced by cold pressing.

Florasols or Phytonic Process

Florasol or phytol process is the newest method used in extracting essential oils by utilizing non-CFS (non-chlorofluorocarbons) as solvents. The oils are called phytols, hence the name of the method it stands for. The unique properties of these solvents were recognized for use in food, aromatherapy, perfume and pharmaceutical industries.

Florasol actually comes from the name of the solvent from which it was taken.

Extraction occurs below surrounding temperature level, so there is no occurrence of degradation of the product. The extraction process also uses selective solvents and produces free flowing clear oil, free of waxes.

WHAT CAN AROMATHERAPY HELP WITH?

Aromatherapy is an alternative medicine that primarily uses natural oils as a means of enhancing one's physical and psychological well-being. Many people consider this alternative therapy as a vital part of their daily life since it produces several health benefits. In fact, some of them are now extending the use of aromatherapy to their pets, specifically dogs.

If you have a dog, then you can use aromatherapy for his benefit. It should be noted that aromatherapy typically works through the senses. Aside from the positive effects that your four-legged family member can receive using the sense of touch when you use oils to treat him, he can also gain benefits from the smell and scents.

Remember that a dog's sense of smell is more sensitive than humans, so it is no longer surprising to see aromatherapy getting more and more popular among dog owners. The good thing about dog aromatherapy is that it is versatile that you can use it in treating different problems and conditions affecting your furry friend.

If using it to treat his condition has never come across your mind, then it is time to consider this alternative treatment. However, remember that while it actually offers a host of benefits for him, note that the effects will still depend on the specific oils used in the whole process. Here are some of the safest oils used in dog aromatherapy and how each one can benefit your pet:

- **Cedar Oil** – Using this oil for aromatherapy is a huge help in repelling pests. It works in killing and controlling fleas, ticks, and other parasites. Combined with other inactive ingredients, cedar wood can offer more relaxing and positive effects to dogs. In addition, it also promotes a healthy skin. It can also help calm him, especially during stressful situations.

- **Lavender Oil** – Used in aromatherapy, this oil has several properties that can benefit your pet. What is good about this oil is that you can use it either diluted or pure. One of its benefits to dogs is its sedative and calming action. It is useful in calming fearful, anxious, hyperactive, and agitated dogs. The oil is versatile enough while also having the ability to create a sense of harmony and peace.

Make it a point to use therapeutic-grade lavender oil for aromatherapy each time your dog faces a stressful situation, such as during a visit to his vet or when you are taking him with you on a trip. It is also useful when you are still training him to quell his hyperactivity. Many dog owners also use lavender oil in aromatherapy for fleas and ticks control. While it does not kill them exactly, it still works in repelling them.

Lavender also has properties designed to relieve some skin conditions affecting your dog, including dryness and itchiness, thereby promoting better skin health. Aside from all the mentioned benefits, lavender also has a scent which is effective in controlling pet odor.

- **Lemongrass Oil** – One of the many things that lemongrass oil can do when used in dog aromatherapy is to control tick and fleas. Even just a small amount of it is enough to produce a citrus smell that dogs often find pleasant but is actually off-putting when inhaled by ticks and fleas. Such is helpful in driving them away. Aside from that, lemongrass oil also improves your dog's skin condition.

- **Eucalyptus Oil** – Eucalyptus is also a popular and safe oil used in dog aromatherapy. Just like lavender and lemongrass, it is effective in controlling fleas and repelling other parasites. It is also good for your dog's skin as it has soothing effects while offering immediate relief to stings, insect bites, and rashes. It has antiseptic and disinfectant properties, too – all of which are useful in dealing with some skin problems.

Furthermore, the oil has inhalant properties that work efficiently in combatting respiratory problems, like bronchitis and sinus infections. If you want to control your pet's odor, then the pleasant smell of the oil can help.

- **Frankincense Oil** – If you want to use a less potent and safer essential oil when applying aromatherapy for dog care, then frankincense oil is the answer. The good thing about frankincense is that it is versatile in the sense that you can use it for a number of functions, including wound care, antibacterial healing, and behavior improvement.

- **Clary Sage Oil** – You can also take advantage of the beneficial properties of this oil to dogs. It works in calming their nerves. Another advantage of clary sage oil is that it works gently, provided you only use small amounts of it and dilute it properly. Doing such works in sedating the central nervous system, thereby calming even the most aggressive dogs.

- **Peppermint Oil** – Another essential oil popularly used in aromatherapy is peppermint. It has become popular because of its numerous benefits including its ability to repel parasites and insects and stimulate circulation. It also helps in treating strains, sprains, dysplasia, and arthritis. If you combine the use of the oil with ginger, then you will have an effective solution for motion sickness.

- **Spearmint Oil** – What is good about this essential oil for aromatherapy is that it aids in managing your dog's weight. It is also beneficial in treating nausea, diarrhea, and colic. In addition, it can balance your dog's metabolism, stimulate the proper functioning of his gallbladder, and prevent gastrointestinal issues.

- **Chamomile Oil** – One thing that makes chamomile oil beneficial for dogs is that it has anti-inflammatory properties that are good for their coat and skin. It also lessens allergic reactions. In addition, it is effective in calming nerves and reducing cramps and muscle and teething pain.

- **Cardamom Oil** – It is a natural diuretic, which also contains anti-bacterial properties. It is ideal for dog aromatherapy as it aids in soothing nausea, treating cough, and normalizing his appetite, especially if he tends to eat less than usual.

The oils used in dog aromatherapy contribute a lot on the benefits that your pet can generate. Aside from the already mentioned positive effects, aromatherapy using safe essential oils can also offer the following:

- Offers an invigorating or sedating effect, thereby promoting relaxation to dogs who easily get nervous and anxious
- Calms aggressive behavior and treats hyperactivity and separation anxiety
- Relieves burns, rashes, and other minor skin irritations, including dog allergies
- Relieves joint problems, including growing pains and arthritis
- Prevents and treats gingivitis and bad breath
- Lessens effects of arthritis
- Combats nausea
- Prevents motion and travel sickness
- Reduces the risk of suffering from coughs, respiratory problems, and congestion

The good thing about dog aromatherapy is that its methods are actually easy to implement. In comparison to pills and medicines that offer negative side effects to your dog, aromatherapy is a more natural treatment, making it safe to use. It benefits not only the dog but you, as the pet owner, too.

For instance, giving him a bath using lavender essential oil also gives you the chance to breathe in the oil's aroma. It can then penetrate into your bloodstream through your respiratory system, which is helpful in soothing and relaxing you.

Some Limitations to Take Note of

It should be noted, though, that while aromatherapy offers numerous benefits to dogs, there are still some limitations to it. That said, you need to get the advice of a veterinarian before using the alternative therapy to your dog. Your veterinarian is skilled enough in diagnosing diseases affecting your dog, so you have to consult him/her, especially during those instances when there are severe or persistent symptoms.

Inform your vet about all the natural products that your dog uses and make him/her a part of your decision. Your vet knows exactly what is good and safe for your dog so listen to him. Also, take note that while essential oils help in affecting mentation and healing, they are also very potent, causing plenty of adverse effects if used incorrectly. One main problem in the essential oils used in aromatherapy is that they are rich in adulterants and contaminants that might trigger serious issues.

With that in mind, you really have to be aware of some precautionary and safety measures before implementing this form of alternative therapy to your dog (more about safety measures in the next section of this book). Furthermore, you need to ensure that he is in perfect condition. Make sure that he is not suffering from any health problem that might negatively interact with the oil you are planning to use.

Furthermore, avoid using the therapy for very young or old puppies, as well as for nursing pups and pregnant dogs. Consult your veterinarian first prior to using any treatment, whether it is natural or otherwise.

Overall, dog aromatherapy is one of those forms of treatments designed to help you take good care of your pet. It offers a solid support to the usual traditional veterinary medicine. There are even instances when the therapy replaces the latter. However, you need to be fully aware of how it works. It is also important to gain a full understanding of how certain essential oils affect dogs prior to using them.

The next section of this book will focus more on some precautionary measures that you can apply when using dog aromatherapy just to make sure that your dog stays safe during the whole procedure.

SAFETY MEASURES BEFORE USING ESSENTIAL OILS WITH YOUR DOGS

While essential oils are generally known for being safe and natural, they still have some adverse effects when used incorrectly. If it is your first time to implement dog aromatherapy, then take note that the key to its success is picking the right and safest essential oil and using it correctly. That way, you no longer have to think about the oil causing negative reactions. It should also be noted that in comparison to humans, dogs have a much more acute sense of smell. They have more than 2 million scent receptors present in their nasal passages, making their sense of smell around 10,000-

100,000 times more acute than human beings.

They can detect odors in part per trillion. This means that while it is possible for you to detect that your cup of coffee contains one teaspoon of sugar, your dog can detect one teaspoon of sugar in one million gallons of water. Your dog makes use of his strong sense of smell to generate all forms of information, no matter how complex these are, from their present environment.

They then take advantage of such information to predict and calculate the states of energy and the perfect response for a specific situation. Due to their strong sense of smell, you can expect them to inhale the scent of essential oils rapidly. The scent can then pass via their bloodstream quickly, making aromatherapy one of the most efficient and fast-acting solutions to treating various conditions affecting dogs.

The problem with your dog's strong sense of smell is that it might also cause them to ingest scents and other properties present in certain essential oils that are actually harmful to them. With that in mind, you really have to learn more about essential oils, how to use them safely for dog aromatherapy, and ensure that you are using just enough for his well-being.

The Truth about Essential Oils

Essential oils are actually volatile substances present in glandular hairs, veins, or sacs of various parts of plants, like their bark, flowers, leaves, fruits, roots, and seeds. They are responsible for the unique scents of different plants. Contrary to what a lot of people believe, they are not actually oily. In fact, they are highly concentrated, which is one of the reasons why you need to dilute them prior to each use. Each essential oil also comes with its unique properties, including color, scent, healing effects, and chemical properties.

Since the oils are highly concentrated, they are also extremely potent. That said, you need to be careful when using them to your dogs. Avoid overusing the oils. In addition, it is important to dilute them with a carrier oil, like sweet almond or olive oil, prior to each use. Make sure to look for aromatherapy oils known for their safe effects on dogs, too. They should be in their diluted forms when used so you can safely use them for your dogs and guarantee positive therapeutic effects.

Also, take note that each pet is different, so expect different reactions depending on the essential oil you used and the specific application method you followed. While most of these essential oils are generally safe for dogs, there are certain types that you need to use carefully or avoid completely.

If you are also a cat owner, then you have to be even more cautious when using certain essential oils. It is mainly because cats are sensitive to oils with polyphenolic compounds. Such compounds can negatively interfere with proper liver detoxification.

Assessing the Quality of the Essential Oils

To guarantee the safety of your dog, ensure that you invest in high-quality essential oils. Note that there are low-quality ones out there that contain lots of harmful and toxic chemicals and substances. Check whether the essential oils you are planning to buy are of top-notch quality with the aid of these guidelines:

- **Be wary of low-priced oils** – Do not go for essential oils offered at extremely low prices as there is a chance that they are low in quality. Go for a reasonably priced brand, which already established a good reputation in the industry. Also, take note that most high-quality essential oils are expensive, so avoid unreasonably low-priced ones as there is a chance that they are also adulterated. Avoid buying the oils at health food stores or supermarkets, too. While they are cheaper, most of them are of low quality.

- **Choose organic oil** – Buying an organic variety is crucial in preventing the risk of pesticide contamination. The majority of brands actually carry the official seal of USDA, but it is important to find an oil, which has the word "wild-crafted" on its label. This means that the oil was created using a plant harvested in the wild. The plant is not farmed, meaning it does not contain chemicals sprayed by farmers.

- **Check if the label indicates that it is 100% pure** – If it does not have such phrase in the label, then there is a great chance that it is altered. There is also a chance that another ingredient is used in it. If you want to use an essential oil, which can really improve the health and well-being of your dog, then make sure that it is pure and does not contain any unwanted and unnecessary chemicals and substances. Another sign that you are getting a high-quality and pure essential oil is if it is in cobalt, violet, or amber glass bottles.

- **Look for vital information about the oils** – You can find the information on the label, in the brochure, or the store's official website. Some of the information you have to find are its Latin name, common name, method of extraction, country of origin and cultivation method – ex. cultivated, organic, and wild-harvested. There should also be 100% pure essential oil printed on its label.

If you have a hard time finding such details from the store's provided resources, including its label, then consider this as a red flag. The provider of the product should make it easy for you to obtain some important information about the oils.

Some Safety and Precautionary Measures

Aside from learning about the essential oils that you should avoid as well as how to assess their quality, you also have to take note of some safety and precautionary measures when using them for dog aromatherapy.

1. *Use high-quality, therapeutic-grade oils* – These are the safest oils that you can use for dogs. Low quality ones often contain additives while being stretched by adding multiple carrier oils, leading to pet sensitivities. There are also low quality ones made by combining oils with other absolutes or botanicals resembling certain scents. They are actually unhealthy not only for your dog but also for you because they contain solvents.

That said, make sure to choose pure and therapeutic brands of essential oils offered by reputable companies. Use the guidelines mentioned earlier to assess their quality. Ensure that they do not contain any added chemicals, too. If you want your dog to ingest the oils directly, the labels should indicate that they are indeed "for internal use". If you can avoid it, though, do not let your dog ingest the oils directly as doing so might harm him. Check the labels, too, to determine if there are clear instructions in diluting the oils, ensuring their proper and safe use.

2. *Dilute the essential oils* – Excess use of the oils might lead to liver failure and might also trigger skin irritation. If you use undiluted ones, then there is a tendency for your pet's sensitive sense of smell

to be affected. Dogs' sense of smell are more sensitive when compared to humans, so diluting the oils even if you just want your pet to inhale them is important in addressing common concerns related to safety.

To dilute, a rough guide is to mix around 3-6 drops of your chosen essential oils to 30-ml or 1-ounce carrier oil. Some of the carrier oils that are safe for this purpose are olive, sweet almond and jojoba oil. If you are still a beginner in using aromatherapy oils, then consider doing a patch test first to check for allergies or sensitivities.

Do this by applying a small drop of the oil you are planning to use on a concealed area. A good place is the skin found on the upper inner part of his leg. Leave it for 24 hours then check again to find out of there is any irritation, redness or swelling.

3. *Use a high-quality aromatherapy diffuser* – As has been mentioned earlier, dogs have a strong sense of smell, so the common mistake committed by pet owners is using the oil excessively. To avoid such mistake, make it a point to use a high-quality aromatherapy diffuser. With the help of this diffuser, you will have full control over the amount of emitted oil. Look for a high-quality diffuser as it can help diffuse just the right amount into the air, thereby preventing you and your dog from getting too overwhelmed with the scent and its effects.

4. *Test the oil's purity* – Before using the essential oil, you need to have a guarantee that it is 100% pure. Even if the label indicates that it is pure, you have to be sure by testing its purity right after you purchase it. You can do this test by putting one drop of the oil into a piece of paper. Let it dry. You will instantly know that the oil is not pure if it leaves behind an oil ring into the white paper.

Note, though, that there are certain exceptions to this rule. It is because there are certain oils that are heavier in terms of consistency and deeper in color – ex. German chamomile, patchouli oils, and sandalwood. Such might still leave some tint behind. In this case, your goal should be to check if the tint is greasy as the grease signifies that it is not pure.

5. *Use the aromatherapy oils only to address a concern affecting your dog and not as a means of preventing a specific health condition* – For instance, avoid letting your dog inhale the oil after eating even if you know that he does not have a digestive problem. Dog aromatherapy is not meant to treat a problem which is not yet there.

6. *Consult your veterinarian* – Before using any oil, ask your vet about it first. Find out if it is really safe to use for your dog. You need a vet's advice especially if he is below ten weeks old, pregnant, or has an existing medical condition. It is also important to consult him regarding the proper use of the oil based on the breed, size, health history, and age.

7. *Consider the size of your dog* – If he is small, then he is more prone to experiencing the usual harmful side effects of the oil, so consider using or applying only a small

amount. When diluting, take into consideration his actual size. Also, avoid using the oils on puppies below eight weeks old who come from medium to large breed. If you have a small breed puppy, however, then you can safely use the oils but make sure that he is already at least ten weeks. That's the safest time for you to apply the oils.

8. *Introduce the oils in a positive environment* – What you can do is to let him smell it first then wait for a while to check for signs of acceptance. Some signs that will let you know that your dog accepts the oils are when he rubs himself against you and when he wants to lick the oil. If there is a positive response, then you can apply the oil. However, if you notice that he turns his head away or do some other things, like whining, sneezing, pacing, drooling, or panting, then it signifies that he does not like the oil, so you need to use a different one.

9. *Do not use the essential oils on sensitive areas* – Some of the areas where you should avoid applying the diluted oil into are the genitals, anal area, eyes and nose. You actually have no reason to put it on the mentioned areas, so avoid doing so as much as possible if you do not want your dog to feel extremely uncomfortable.

Probably the most important among the tips already mentioned is to avoid adding the essential oil to your dog's drinking water or food. Any form of direct ingestion should be avoided as it is not meant for that purpose. Use the other aromatherapy applications that we will discuss later instead of direct ingestion.

IS AROMATHERAPY SUITABLE FOR YOUR DOG?

Just like how useful aromatherapy is for humans, it is also beneficial for pets, especially dogs who need healing because of its therapeutic and positive emotional effects. With the therapy's increasing number of benefits, it is no longer surprising to see it as a popular alternative healing technique designed to cure a variety of health-related and emotional issues affecting dogs. It is designed to deal with emotional disorders and physical diseases.

If your dog lives indoors, then he might have already lost his primal abilities. In most cases, dogs who freely roam outdoors look happier because they have the opportunity to run around and do what they want the entire day However, they also spend their day smelling almost all kinds of things, particularly those that are in their purest and most natural form. Letting them sniff and smell the beneficial aromatherapy oils is a big help in healing any physical and emotional disorders that they have.

The question now is whether or not aromatherapy oils are really suitable for your dog. You don't want to put his health condition at risk, do you? So there is a chance that you would want to conduct an extensive research first prior to exposing him to any essential oil. Note that while aromatherapy makes use of essential oils designed to produce scents enjoyed by humans, there are also volatile substances and compounds present in the oils, making them potentially toxic when used to your dog at specific concentrations.

Also, take note that dogs are sensitive to these essential oils. With that in mind, you will realize that what is actually safe for people does not necessarily mean that it is safe for your dog, too. Not applying it correctly and on the right place might cause your dog to inhale, eat, or lick the oils inadvertently. There is also a chance for his skin to absorb the oils.

Since dogs react differently when exposed to these substances, it is essential to discuss your plan to use aromatherapy oils with your vet and listen to what he has to say about it. Make sure that your furry friend won't really experience pain, discomfort, or other health issues due to it.

Are Aromatherapy Oils Safe for your Dog?

Generally, all dog breeds can safely use aromatherapy oils. However, you have to take extreme caution especially if he is from a breed that is prone to or has existing breathing problems. Some dog breeds that commonly suffer from breathing problems, like brachycephalic airway syndrome, are pug, boxer, bulldog, Shih Tzu, Staffordshire bull terrier, Boston terrier, and Pekingese. If your dog is from any of the mentioned breeds, then be extra cautious in implementing any of the aromatherapy methods.

Talk to your vet first and ask for a

professional opinion to determine if it is safe to use aromatherapy and the corresponding essential oils even if your pet is prone to breathing problems or difficulties. Also, keep in mind that while the majority of dogs have less or zero problems when it comes to using essential oils, you need to be extra careful if you are still new to using this alternative therapy to dogs.

As a rule of thumb, puppies who are from medium to large breeds, like the German shepherd, Labrador retriever, Otter hound, and Saint Bernard, who are not yet 10 weeks of age should never be exposed to aromatherapy oils. It is because the substances are not yet safe for puppies of the mentioned breeds who are around that age. Wait for them to reach ten weeks before starting to implement aromatherapy.

Another rule to keep in mind is to avoid using the oils on toy dogs, as well as pregnant and old ones. It is mainly because these are among the most sensitive types of pets, requiring additional care. You can't expose them to certain elements and substances that may only have a negative impact on their overall health. Aromatherapy oil is not suitable for epileptic dogs, too.

How to Determine if an Essential Oil is Safe for your Dog?

Animals, especially dogs, metabolize and react in a much different way to essential oils than humans, so it is crucial to know about such differences to avoid any negative reactions. One common problem encountered is overusing the oils. There are instances when dog owners diffuse too much oils into their households, causing unintentional overdose for dogs. You can avoid this from happening by testing your dog's reaction to the oil first and figuring out the safest dose for him.

Fortunately, there are a few tests designed to help you determine the suitability and safety of an essential oil for dogs. For instance, if your dog has never smelled any natural or essential oil in the past, then let him sniff your chosen mixture first and observe his initial reaction. If he responds negatively, then it may not be the best and safest oil for him. However, it is still possible for you to make him get used to the smell.

What you have to do is to place the aromatherapy oil in a diluted mist form. Spray a bit of it in the place where he sleeps and usually roam around. That way, he can start getting used to the smell. If you can't still get him to like the oil, then maybe it is not really suitable for him so it is advisable to look for another one, which he can easily adopt.

If your pet is sensitive, then make sure to check for any signs of negative reaction. Use small doses first. Avoid using your chosen oil at full strength if it is still the first time for your dog to get exposed to it.

Another tip is to pre-select around three to five essential oils from the ones known to be safe for them. Make sure that your choice also depends on the specific issue that you want to address. Pre-selecting at least three beneficial oils will let you choose one, which your dog particularly likes and is suitable for his specific condition and needs.

Once you have made the selection, offer each oil to him one at a time. Each one should still be in a closed bottle when you offer it to your dog. Let him sniff the bottle while it is closed. Keep in mind that with your dog's excellent sense of smell, he can sniff the scent even if it is closed.

Observe his reaction so you will know which one he really likes. Some of the signs and reactions to watch out for that might indicate that the oil does not suit your dog are nervousness, whining, and excessive scratching. Once you determined the oil preferred by your dog, dilute it accordingly. You can then start offering it to him again through inhalation.

Also, ensure that you use oils that are safe and suitable for most dogs. Keep in mind that there are those that are not suitable for them, posing dangers especially when used in extremely large amounts. Avoid using the following essential oils, too, as they are not safe for dogs and might only trigger skin sensitivities, allergies, and interference to their natural body functions.

- **Camphor, White Thyme, Juniper, Yarrow and Anise** – All these oils can trigger possible toxicity or uterine stimulation, so avoid using them on your dog, especially if pregnant ones. As for juniper, you can actually use the juniper berry oil variety as it is safe for dogs. However, do not use juniper wood oil as it is toxic to the kidneys.

- **Wintergreen and Birch** – While you can actually use these aromatherapy oils for joint pains and arthritis, it is not ideal for dermal or skin purposes. It is because of their toxic properties caused by the high methyl salicylate content. Ensure that your dog does not ingest it in any way, too, as it might lead to severe poisoning, and even death.

- **Clove Leaf and Bud** – Avoid these oils, too, because these tend to trigger dermal irritation. They can also lead to toxicity not only to your dog but also to you and the people around.

- **Horseradish and Mustard** – Both of these oils have pungent properties, making them risky when used on dogs. They may also trigger severe dermal irritation.

- **Wormwood** – Wormwood is toxic to pets, particularly dogs, so make sure to avoid it as much as possible. It triggers seizures while also holding high dermal and oral toxicity.

- **Oregano** – It is a toxic oil for dogs so avoid using it as much as possible. However, there are still instances when you can use it but only in extremely small amounts and after you diluted it properly with a carrier oil. Such results to an aromatherapy solution, which is good for dogs who have poor respiratory health. Despite that, it is important for you to spend time weighing all the risks involved in applying the oregano oil. Also, consider vital factors, like your dog's breed, size, and age, and discuss this with your vet first.

- **Tea Tree** – Tea tree oil can also put your dog at risk, especially if you use extremely high doses. It is still beneficial but only in small amounts. Ensure that your dog does not have too much contact with tea tree.

Make it a point to use other essential oils in dog aromatherapy, instead of the ones mentioned above, to guarantee his safety. Note that while aromatherapy for dogs is extremely beneficial for his overall health, there are also risks if you choose to apply one, which is not suitable for him.

Typical Safety Precautions When Using Essential Oils on Canines

- Use essential oils that are safe and 100 percent pure on dogs and humans.
- Be sure to dilute essential oils before using on dogs. For a rough guide, add 5-6 drops of essential oil to 1 ounce or 30 ml. of carrier base oil. For 8 ounces or 240 ml. of shampoo, use 20-25 drops of essential oils.
- Use smaller amounts of diluted oil on smaller dogs, puppies and aged dogs whose health is compromised. If you are not sure if your dog's current condition can take essential oils, then start off with hydrosols.
- Never use essential oils on dogs with epilepsy or who are prone to seizure attacks. Some oils such as rosemary can trigger seizures even in humans.

- Avoid applying essential oils around the eyes, or close to the nose, anal or genital organs. These areas contain easily irritated membranes and can be susceptible to increased chemical absorption.
- Do not fail to check with a holistic veterinarian before using any essential oils on pregnant dogs. Essential oils like peppermint, eucalyptus, tea tree and rosemary must be avoided especially when your dog is pregnant.
- Some oils are not suitable for use on dogs ever, in any quantity. Phenols, such as those in Oregano and Thyme oils are not indicated for use on canines. Pennyroyal and Wormwood oils should never be used. Be sure to only use recipes that you trust, from sources that are educated in aromatherapy and holistic veterinarian practice.

- If your animal has a history of sensitive skin, be sure to patch test any topical treatment on a small area of skin before applying fully. The skin is a complicated organ and it can be hard to predict its reaction. A patch test is the safest way to prevent a large and possibly painful amount of irritation.
- Some oils can increase sensitivity to sunlight. Citrus oils, in particular, are known for this. On short-haired breeds especially, it is very important to make sure your dog's skin is not exposed to these oils and sunlight at the same time. Doing so can increase the risk of sunburn, possibly to a large degree. Ears are a particular area of concern, because in many breeds they tend to be sunlight sensitive to begin with.
- Never assume that an oil that is safe in one application is safe in another.

Some oils are therapeutic when applied topically but useless or, even worse, toxic if taken internally. This is why it is important to follow recipe and application instructions very carefully. Not only that, but make sure the source of your recipe is a trusted and educated source.

- Always make sure your supply of essential oils, carrier oils and mixtures made with them are stored properly. Above all: they must be stored out of the reach of your animals. Some oils can smell quite tasty to dogs, but if they are ingested in any but the smallest quantities they are toxic. Even a neutral oil like vegetable oil will cause digestive troubles if eaten in large amounts. Treat these ingredients and remedies as you would any other medicine by making sure there is no way your dog can access them. If you ever suspect that your dog has obtained access to them, monitor them very closely for symptoms and call your veterinarian.

- Tea Tree oil is a common home remedy for bacterial issues. However, it can be too strong for dogs, especially small ones. If you do decide to use it, be cautious at first, always do a patch test and limit the duration of exposure. Also consider that you may be able to swap Sweet Marjoram oil for it and still achieve the desired effect.
- "Hot spots" like at the joint of the legs or neck may be more sensitive to topical applications than the spine or sides would be. On animals with a lot of fur or skin, keep in mind that where the skin meets skin or stays much warmer, it can intensify the effect of the oil. If it is necessary to apply remedies to these areas, keep in mind that it may be advisable to dilute the

mixture to account for this. A patch test is helpful in this instance as well.

- When using a diffuser to disperse essential oils in your home there are a few precautions that will make it safer. First, turn diffusers off when you aren't at home. Dogs are more sensitive to smells than we are, so without being able to see and monitor your pet, there is no way to know if the scent has become too strong. Secondly, keep your diffuser clean. If it becomes contaminated with dust, mold or other particulate matter, those will be diffused through your home as well. This can cause all sorts of irritation and problems and is very easy to avoid.

- Consider carrier oils carefully. Depending on your dog's skin and where the mixture is being applied, you may see a range of reactions. With a patch test, for instance, you may see dryness or slight irritation. Sometimes this is not due to the essential oil at all, but to the carrier oil. Oils like Avocado or Coconut may simply be too heavy for your animal's particular skin and fur needs. Conversely, mildly astringent oils like Mint or Rosemary may cause irritation when blended with a very lightweight oil like Apricot Seed, but could be perfect when carried in something richer. If skin sensitivity is a concern, patch test all carrier oils on their own so you can see how your dog reacts before mixing other essential oils in.

DIFFERENT AROMATHERPY APPLICATIONS

Due to the many benefits of essential oils, it is safe to say that these serve as powerful tools in the health care toolkit of your dogs. Using them properly and correctly in aromatherapy can help you deal with the most common concerns affecting dogs, including anxiety and stress. The good thing about aromatherapy oils is that they are natural. This means that you can improve the health condition of your dog without sedation or intense drugs. All that you need is the natural soothing power provided by the aromatherapy oils.

Even small amounts of the oils can already help in treating a host of health conditions and problems. It heals the entire body – both physically and emotionally. In addition, the oils contain plenty of antiseptic, revitalizing, detoxifying, regulating, anti-microbial, and calming properties, making them truly valuable for both humans and dogs.

However, it is important to understand how to use and apply it properly. Used correctly, the oils serve as gentle, safe, and natural solutions for treating various dog problems without any side effects. Aromatherapy serves as a great solution for allergies, fear, anxiety, liver function, joint problems, skin conditions, and other issues that hamper the overall health condition of your dog.

The Different Application Methods

You have a few options when it comes to applying the aromatherapy oils into your dog. Just make sure that whichever method you choose, you prioritize his safety. Here are some of the ways for you to apply the oils on your dog safely and ensure that he will get all the benefits promised by aromatherapy.

1. **Massage** – Prior to massaging your chosen oil into his skin, dilute it first. Dilute it in a base oil before massaging on the affected area. Once in the diluted form, you can gently massage it into a hairless part of your dog's skin, like the inner thigh, groin, or armpit. You can also go to the part with the least amount of hair. Do this for around three to four minutes.

If you choose to apply the aromatherapy oils directly into his skin through a gentle massage, then a wise tip is to only cover those areas starting from his neck to his tail. Choose oils that can quickly penetrate into his skin, too, so he can start enjoying the effects as soon as possible. However, you need to avoid applying the oil directly or close to his face, nose, or eyes. Prevent it from getting ingested internally, too.

In this case, be careful when massaging the oil. Make it a point to put the oil in a part of his body where he can't lick. However, even if the massage application only involves applying the oil externally, you should still avoid doing it if your dog is pregnant or prone to seizures. Only do it once you receive the go-signal of your vet.

2. **Diffuser** – You can also try aromatherapy for dogs using a diffuser. In this case, you need to combine your chosen aromatherapy oil with a source of heat. The good news is that you have plenty of options when it comes to using a diffuser for dog aromatherapy.

   For instance, you can go for those diffusers that operate using electricity. There are also those that require candles. Another option is a ring-shaped device, which you need to place on the topmost part of a light bulb. To use your chosen diffuser, follow these guidelines:

   - Place the recommended number of drops of your chosen essential oil into the diffuser. Doing this will prompt the scents of the aromatherapy oil to instantly fill up the room.

- Let your dog stay in the room filled up with the scent for around thirty minutes. This will allow him to breathe in the oil as it evaporates into the air.

- To guarantee better results, consider doing this two times daily. Done properly, it is possible for you to see positive results within 5-7 days.

If you decide to use a diffuser, though, ensure that your dog has an escape route just in case he does not like the scent produced by the oil. With an escape route, he can easily get out of the room right away if he starts to feel uncomfortable.

3. **Topical application** – This is a popular way to use aromatherapy for dogs. In this form of application, you will need to apply your chosen oil directly into the

needed area/s. Such will let the oil penetrate deeply into the skin. The small capillaries will then absorb it quickly, carrying the oils into the bloodstream. You can actually apply your chosen aromatherapy oil to your dog topically via massage, which has already been explained earlier.

Another way to apply it topically is with the help of sprays or spritzers. You also have the option to put it on dog shampoo, conditioner, ointment, or salve and apply it to your pet topically using the mentioned products. Diluting the oil should be the first thing you have to do before using it topically. In this case, you can make use of carrier oils, including sweet almond, jojoba, or olive oil.

4. **Petting** – If you want a less intense topical application of aromatherapy oil to your dog, then petting is an ideal option. What you have to do is to place the diluted oil into your hands. Rub your hands containing the oil until

it produces a light film based on your preferred concentration.

Use both your hands to pet the dog with the oil. This is a less intense technique of using aromatherapy to address common emotional issues affecting dogs, like depression, stress, and anxiety. Petting and the diluted oil both work in calming him down.

Regardless of which method you choose, make sure to use a high-quality essential oil for it. Also, remember not to be tempted to put the oil into his food nor rub it on him even if you noticed that he does not want it. Avoid forcing the oil on him as doing so might cause adverse reactions. Use only those aromatherapy oils that draw a positive response from him.

Basic Rules Before the Final Application

To ensure that you apply the aromatherapy oils correctly using any of the approaches mentioned above, you have to be fully aware of the basic rules involved in it. One is to decide on the specific oil that should help your dog first. What you have to do is to create a shortlist of at least five aromatherapy oils. Put each one in a closed bottle then let each settle on your floor with enough spaces in between.

Encourage your dog to come close to the bottles and smell them. Observe and figure out which one among the closed bottles he sniffs intently or in some cases, tries to lick. Your dog will most likely stop sniffing once he finally reached the oil he wants and needs. Let him make the choice as he actually has the ability to pick exactly the one he needs. Note that each dog has the ability to pick the exact oil required for his condition, so give him a chance to guide his own healing through this activity.

Make sure that you fully understand a dog's major responses to the oils, too. In most cases, dogs use three major ways to respond to the aromatic extracts. These are smelling/inhalation, localized topical application, and licking. Inhalation is considered to be the most powerful because the oils tend to go directly to the brain using the dog's olfactory system, which then alters his brain chemistry.

In most cases, your dog will also show you what he wants you to do with the oil by pointing his head into a specific part of his body, moving into you, or stamping his foot. If he does any of these, then note that he might want you to apply the oil on a specific part of his body topically, usually in an acupuncture point. When this happens, just rub a small amount of the oil into the indicated body part.

Diluting the Oil

After choosing a specific oil, diluting it should follow. This is an important step you should not neglect as the undiluted form may be too strong and powerful for your dog to handle. If you use too much of the oil in its undiluted form, then your dog might deal with adverse reactions, such as skin irritation and liver failure. You can dilute it by mixing around 1-3 drops of the oil in a teaspoon of cold-pressed vegetable oil – ex. olive or sunflower oil. Once diluted, you can offer it to your dog then observe how he responds to it.

If there is a positive response, then you

can start offering this to him based on your chosen application one to two times daily. Do this routine until he starts losing interest in the oil. There is a chance for him to lose interest in the diluted oil within 3 days to one week. If this happens, you will also notice a significant change in the problem you are planning to treat.

If you have young pups, old dogs, or those who are sick causing them to require special care and attention, then avoid giving them too much of the oil. Note that increasing the dosage won't be of help at all in the mentioned cases. In fact, if you are still in doubt, a wise advice is to use lesser amount of the diluted oil than what is recommended. You can also utilize a diffuser initially just to be safe.

Despite being in their diluted form, you have to take note that the essential oils are strong, so you should avoid direct contact to your dog's eye area, inner ear, or face. If you plan to use it on his tummy, then focus on what you are doing to avoid the risk of the oil reaching his anal or genital area.

Consider your Dog Breed's Size

Before the final application, keep in mind that the size of your dog contributes a lot on the specific amount of essential oil you need to use. If you have a small dog breed, then three to five drops are already more than enough. Dilute around 80 to 90% of it before application. If you have large dogs, then begin with three to five drops. In this case, you can use the undiluted oils unless the product label instructs you to do otherwise.

For giant dog breeds, like a Great Dane, you can still give them diluted essential oils but consider increasing the dosage - at least 6 drops will do. For very small pups, such as a tiny Yorkie, around 1-2 drops are often enough. You need to avoid overdosing your dog with the oil, so be extra cautious when applying the products.

AROMATHERAPY TOOLS AND MATERIALS

For you to start taking full advantage of aromatherapy for dogs, you need to gather a few tools and materials. This chapter will talk about everything that you will most likely need once you decide to introduce aromatherapy oils to your dog. If you have all these tools and materials, then making the most out of the oils in terms of improving your dog's health is possible.

Essential Oils

Of course, you need a collection of essential oils known to be safe for dogs. You can refer to a previous chapter of this book to determine which oils are safe to use for pets, especially dogs, and which ones are not. Before making your choice out of the many essential oils today, have a vet check your dog first to figure out if the one you intend to use is safe for him.

Such is crucial in determining if he has an undiagnosed health problem that might negatively react to the procedure. Also, if you want to make a more modest investment with essential oils, consider purchasing those in 5-ml bottles first. Take note of some of the most expensive varieties, like the Frankincense and chamomile, and determine if you are willing to shell out more money for them.

Carrier Oils

Carrier oils are also among the most important items you need before you can start taking advantage of aromatherapy for dogs. In fact, they serve as the foundation of the majority of blends. You can use them in diluting the essential oils so they will be safe to apply on your dog's skin.

With a good collection of safe carrier oils, you can produce diluted forms of the essential oils that you can safely distribute to the different parts of your dog's body. Some of the best carrier oils that are suitable for dog aromatherapy are olive, coconut, sunflower, apricot, grape seed, and sweet almond oil.

Measuring Spoons and Cups

Once you decide to make your own aromatherapy blends for dogs, it is necessary for you to invest in a separate set of measuring spoons and cups from the ones in your kitchen. Make sure to use these items only for the purpose of measuring ingredients for the blends. As mentioned in some parts of this book, dogs are sensitive. They have a strong sense of smell.

With that in mind, you have to make sure that your blends have the right amount of essential and carrier oils, as well as other ingredients. Inaccurate measurement might lead to producing aromatherapy blends that might harm your dog, instead of healing him.

If you plan to measure large quantities, then it would be best to have a Pyrex measuring cup, which also comes with a pour spout. Your measuring spoon also plays a major role as you can use it to measure essential oils accurately, especially if you need more than just a few drops.

Bottles/Containers

Bottles and other containers should also form part of the tools you own for aromatherapy. A few bottles, jars, and other containers are crucial if you want to store your produced blend properly. Some bottles and containers that you can use for the safe storage of the blends are the following:

- *Amber Glass Bottle* – Consider getting one with a secure lid. You can also go for amber glass bottles with droppers as these promote ease in adding the correct number of drops needed for a specific situation. Make sure to go for nice bottles that are dark enough to ensure that the blends inside are protected while still allowing you to see exactly what is inside and how much is already left.

- *Glass Roller Bottle* – A glass roller bottle is also another of those supplies that you will love to have on hand for use in dog aromatherapy. You can go for small 10-ml bottles that have roller ball tops in producing your own blends. With the roller top, you can easily apply the aromatherapy blends to your dog then store the bottle somewhere safe once you are done using it.

- *Glass Spray Bottle* – You can also make use of this specific container if you plan to take advantage of aromatherapy for dogs through inhalation. You just need to put your created blends in this bottle then spray some in a room where your dog often stays.

No matter what type of bottles or containers you use for storing your produced aromatherapy blends, ensure that they are securely covered. Also, make sure that they are made of materials and come in colors that will let you clearly see what is inside. It is also advisable to label each container. Put the exact date you made it, the ingredients, name of the blend, or any other important details in the label. That way, you won't end up using the wrong one for your dog.

Diffuser

It is also essential for you to invest in a good quality diffuser. Note that diffusing essential oils into the air, especially if your dog is in an enclosed space, such as a room in your house or his kennel, is one of the most effective applications of aromatherapy for dogs. Such allows the sweet-smelling and highly aromatic molecules of essential oils to be breathed in by the dogs, stimulating several healing, stimulation, relaxation, and immune-boosting responses.

The good thing about having a high-quality diffuser is that it lets you diffuse oil into the kennel or your home, which aids in naturally purifying air by getting rid of toxins, harmful microscopic debris, and metallic particles. It also inhibits the reproduction and growth of airborne pathogens, letting you and your pet stay in a safe and healthy environment. The following are just some of the types of diffusers that are suitable for dog aromatherapy:

- *Cold Air Diffuser* – This type of diffuser utilizes room temperature air as a means of blowing your chosen oil into the nebulizer. The goal is to vaporize the oil into the air. What makes this type of diffuser useful is that it works quickly and efficiently. However, it is not that effective in diffusing thicker and heavier essential oils. Many also find it a bit difficult to clean.

- *Evaporative Diffuser* – Another choice is the evaporative diffuser. It has a basic operation, which involves the use of a fan as a means of blowing air through a filter or pad where you put the oil. Such works in vaporizing the oil that you placed in the pad. This diffuser also covers glass pendants, inhalers, and clay pendants.

  There is a drawback, though, such as the fact that it tends to diffuse lighter oils, like citrus, faster than heavier ones. It is more suitable for use when you and your dog are inside your vehicle or during those times when you bring him on a trip.

- *Heat Diffuser* – This is the perfect choice for you if you want to spread a pleasant smell around your home. It aids in producing a nice smell that can soothe or relax your dog. However, if you want to take full advantage of the therapeutic and healing properties present in essential oils, then it would be best to stay away from heat diffuser.

It is because heat has the tendency of changing the oil's properties and chemistries. It can then result to removing the therapeutic and healing properties it has. It would be best to use this diffuser if your goal is just to make your entire home or the specific area your dog is staying in smell more pleasantly.

- *Ultrasonic Diffuser* – This is the best choice especially if you want to make the most out of all the therapeutic benefits and healing properties present in your chosen oil. This diffuser utilizes electronic frequencies as a means of creating vibrations in water. Such vibrations will then be brought into the surface where there are floating essential oils.

With the help of the vibrations, the oils will be vaporized, dispersing their scents and properties into the air – that is possible even if you do not use a source of heat. In comparison to heat diffuser, it does not damage the healing properties of the oils you decide to use. It works efficiently in purifying air while also getting rid of any unwanted odor.

Choose one diffuser, which you think is really effective in spreading the therapeutic benefits of the oil and letting your dog enjoy them.

Storage Box or Shelf

Of course, you also need to invest in a storage box or shelf where you can safely store or place your aromatherapy blends for dogs. You can't mix it with all the other stuff present in your home. You need a separate storage place where you can keep them all together so you won't end up mixing things up and using the wrong stuff for your dog.

The best storage box or shelf is one which allows you to store not only your aromatherapy blends but also all the tools and supplies that you need for the procedure.

Aside from the mentioned tools and supplies, it is also advisable to have a good reference guide or book. This is important especially if you are still a beginner in using aromatherapy for dogs. Even if you are still a beginner, you will feel more at ease with the right reference guide around as you know that you are well-guided in terms of proper use, how to blend certain ingredients, dilution ratios, and other important stuff.

3 GREAT AROMATHERAPIES FOR YOUR DOG

In the last section of this book, you will get to know about three of the best aromatherapy recipes that you can use for your dog and some bonus recipes/blends. The good thing about the recipes here is that they are designed in such a way that they can treat or deal with a number of conditions affecting your dog.

For Easily Stressed, Anxious, and Fearful Dogs

If you have a dog who tends to get easily stressed and anxious, then the aromatherapy blend below will definitely help him. Note that just like humans, dogs are also prone to experiencing some negative emotions, like separation anxiety, fear, nervousness, and stress.

The good news is that you can now address the mentioned issues with the help of therapeutic-grade essential oils. The following recipe is designed to calm and soothe dogs, ensuring that he does not get too stressed out, anxious or fearful in certain situations.

Ingredients:

- 300-ml water
- 5 to 10 drops Roman chamomile essential oil
- 5 to 10 drops lavender essential oil

Instructions:

1. Combine all the ingredients in a bowl. Pour the mixture in a spray bottle. Shake it to mix everything well.

2. Cover the eyes and face of your dog. You can use your hand or a clean cloth as cover and prevent the oil from penetrating the mentioned areas.

3. Spray a light mist around your dog in those instances when he gets anxious, stressed out, or nervous. It can help settle him down. Another option is spraying a mist into your palms then applying the blend through massage. Massage his back, chest, and neck as it can calm him down.

Another variation of the recipe is to use 5 drops each of cedar wood and lavender and mix them in the same amount of water mentioned earlier before putting the blend in a spray bottle. Follow the same instructions above when applying it to your dog. You can also use a diffuser but you have to reduce the amount of essential oils needed.

You can just use one drop of cedar wood, lavender or the chamomile, put enough water in the diffuser then pour the oil into it. Turn the diffuser on to calm your anxious, nervous or fearful dog. Expect the result of this recipe and its variations to offer soothing effects in as little as thirty minutes.

The best time to take advantage of this aromatherapy blend for dogs is ten minutes before you leave home or before the arrival of your guests.

For Flea & Tick Removal

One of the most common issues affecting dogs that aromatherapy oils can treat is the presence of fleas and ticks. Fortunately, it is not that hard to create a recipe designed to remove fleas and ticks and ensure that your dog will no longer deal with the side effects of having them around. Here is one simple recipe that you can try to finally get rid of the problem.

Ingredients:

- 1 drop cedar wood
- 5 drops lavender
- 2 drops citronella
- 1 cup water – Consider doubling this amount if you have a dog who is too sensitive to smell.

Instructions:

1. Get a bowl and mix all the mentioned ingredients well with the aid of a wire whisk.

2. Soak cotton bandannas into it. Allow the bandannas to dry naturally in the sun. You can also use it for dog collars. Just make sure to avoid letting the blend get into the plastic parts of the collars. Note that some essential oils tend to degrade the plastic so be careful.

3. After drying the bandana or dog collar, put it around his neck. In case he is too sensitive to smell, then consider tying the bandana or collar to his harness before taking him for walks. Put it in a place away from his nose.

You can also create a spray version of this recipe, which can repel ticks and fleas naturally. You just need 5 drops of lavender, 2 tablespoons carrier oil and 2 drops each of citronella, lemongrass, and cedar wood. A 10 to 12-ounce spray bottle is also essential in storing the blend after mixing them. Go for a bottle with a 16-ounce capacity, though, especially if you noticed that the blend has a strong scent.

Spray it around your dog while avoiding all parts of his face, including the eyes. You can also spray it just around your house. Because your dog has a strong sense of smell, he can definitely pick up the scent of the aromatherapy blend and enjoy its benefits. If you decide to add more oils than what have been mentioned, then consider reducing the number of drops you use, too. Such is crucial in preventing the final scent from becoming too overwhelming for your dog to handle.

For Proper Skin Health and Support

Your dog's skin can also greatly benefit from certain aromatherapy recipes and blends. If your dog is prone to itchiness, dryness, and other skin irritations, then you can make use of essential oils designed to get rid of the problem and promote better skin health. Aromatherapy oils also help in supporting an aging dog's skin, thereby keeping it healthy no matter how old he is. One recipe designed to promote better skin health in dogs is the following:

Ingredients:

- 5 drops lavender

- 2 tablespoons carrier oil – Your options include olive or jojoba oil.

- 3 drops each of frankincense and Roman chamomile

- 3 drops Vitamin E

Instructions:

1. Combine all the mentioned ingredients in a bowl or measuring cup. Once done, pour the mixture into a roller ball bottle or a dropper bottle. Go for glass-based bottles so you can easily check and monitor the content.

2. Put on two to four drops of the blend to your dog's skin. It is a huge help in maintaining the excellent health of the skin of aging dogs. You can also use it for skin patches that are dry as the blend works in adding moisture to the area.

Aside from the three recipes already mentioned, it is also possible for you to create the following at home with the aid of aromatherapy oils – all of these are designed to improve the overall health and well-being of your dog:

1. **Deodorizing Spray** – Consider making this spray at home, especially if your dog often goes outdoors for long hours and comes back home with an unwanted smell. The only things that you need for this are 5-ounce water, 5 drops lavender essential oil, 15 drops purification oil, and a pinch of salt. Mix the oils with the salt first then stir it gently before pouring the mixture to the water. Spray this blend to your dog to guarantee instant odor relief.

2. **Immune-strengthening Spray** – This easy-to-make spray is designed to strengthen the immune system of your dog. All you need are 5 drops each of lavender and frankincense and just enough water to fill up a 12-ounce spray bottle. Just mix the oils then pour it into the bottle filled with water. Seal it with the lid. Spray it on your dog, avoiding any part of his face as much as possible. You can also massage it on certain parts, like his chest, back, and neck.

3. **Muscle Ache Relief** – If you have an active dog, then there is a great chance for him to overdo his activities, causing pains and aches in the joints and muscles. In this case, you can seek the aid of aromatherapy blends. You can mix together 3 drops of lavender, 2 to 3 drops Copaiba, and a tablespoon of carrier oil then pour the mixture in a glass bottle with a roller ball.

   Anytime your dog shows signs of aching or sore muscles, you can just use the blend by rubbing its roller bottle into the affected area. Massage it gently, too. Expect him to obtain muscle ache relief within just ten to fifteen minutes.

With the three major recipes mentioned above and a couple of bonus recipes, it is safe to assume that aromatherapy for dogs can really help your furry friend live a healthy and happy life. Start taking full advantage of the power of aromatherapy as well as the beneficial and healing properties provided by the essential oils used in this technique to keep your dog at the pink of health.

What's good about aromatherapy is that it does not only work for dogs. You can also start researching about how you and your loved ones can benefit from it when it comes to boosting your health.

ABOUT THE AUTHOR

Julie Summers has dedicated her life to holistic and alternative medicine for our loyal companions. Growing up with a Veterinarian for a mother, animals have always been a large part of Julie's life. She started her journey as far back as she can remember, constantly seeking ways to better care for her animal pals.

Julie started to formally train in aromatherapy and acupressure for animals a decade ago. She received her certification in Natural Health for Animals at the University of Natural Health in 2007.

Outside of being an author, she works as a manager at a dog boarding centre. Employing her deep knowledge of alternative treatments has enabled her to provide outstanding results for all of her clients!

www.ingramcontent.com/pod-product-compliance
Lightning Source LLC
Chambersburg PA
CBHW071157240526
45470CB00016BA/131